The National Body Challenge

Success Program

for the Whole Family

Hay House Titles of Related Interest

The National Body Challenge
Success Program
for the Whole Family

Pamela Peeke,
M.D., M.P.H., F.A.C.P.

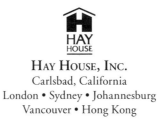

HAY HOUSE, INC.
Carlsbad, California
London • Sydney • Johannesburg
Vancouver • Hong Kong

Published and distributed in the United States by: Hay House, Inc., P.O. Box 5100, Carlsbad, CA 92018-5100 • *Phone:* (760) 431-7695 or (800) 654-5126 • *Fax:* (760) 431-6948 or (800) 650-5115 • www.hayhouse.com • *Published and distributed in Australia by:* Hay House Australia Pty. Ltd., 18/36 Ralph St., Alexandria NSW 2015 • *Phone:* 612-9669-4299 • *Fax:* 612-9669-4144 • www.hayhouse.com.au • *Published and distributed in the United Kingdom by:* Hay House UK, Ltd. • Unit 62, Canalot Studios • 222 Kensal Rd., London W10 5BN • *Phone:* 44-20-8962-1230 • *Fax:* 44-20-8962-1239 • www.hayhouse.co.uk • *Published and distributed in the Republic of South Africa by:* Hay House SA (Pty), Ltd., P.O. Box 990, Witkoppen 2068 • *Phone/Fax:* 27-11-706-6612 • orders@psdprom.co.za • *Distributed in Canada by:* Raincoast • 9050 Shaughnessy St., Vancouver, B.C. V6P 6E5 • *Phone:* (604) 323-7100 • *Fax:* (604) 323-2600

Editorial consultation: Angela Hynes • *Design:* Jeannine Gaubert and Amy Rose Szalkiewicz
Cover and interior photos of Pamela Peeke: Nick Horn • *Stock photos:* www.gettyone.com

The National Body Challenge Success Program Book Development Team: Eileen O'Neill, *General Manager, Discovery Health Channel* • Donald Thoms, *Vice President, Production, Discovery Health Channel* • John Whyte, *Vice President, Continuing Medical Education, Discovery Health Channel* • Sharon M. Bennett, *Senior Vice President, Strategic Partnerships & Licensing* • Michael Malone, *Vice President, Licensing* • Carol LeBlanc, *Vice President, Marketing & Retail Development* • Elizabeth Bakacs, *Vice President, Creative Strategic Partnerships* • Jeannine Gaubert, *Art Director* • Christine Alvarez, *Director of Publishing* • Elsa Abraham, *Publishing Manager* • Erica Rose, *Publishing Associate*

Library of Congress Cataloging-in-Publication Data

Peeke, Pamela.
  The national body challenge success program for the whole family / Pamela Peeke.
    p. cm.
  ISBN-13: 978-1-4019-1049-5 (tradepaper)
  ISBN-10: 1-4019-1049-1 (tradepaper)
  1. Physical fitness. 2. Stress management. 3. Conduct of life. 4. Self-help techniques. 5. Self-esteem. 6. Self-actualization (Psychology) I. Title.
  RA781.P42 2006
  613.7--dc22

                    2005029057

                ISBN 13: 978-1-4019-1049-5
                ISBN 10: 1-4019-1049-1

                08 07 06 05 4 3 2 1
                1st printing, December 2005

        Printed in the United States of America

I dedicate this to every man, woman and child who makes the decision to step up to the plate, take the challenge, and do the work to achieve and then maintain their mental and physical transformation—*for life.*

Contents

PART III: SUCCESS STORIES OF PHYSICAL AND MENTAL TRANSFORMATIONS

Foreword

*by Arkansas Governor Mike Huckabee
and First Lady Janet Huckabee*

Like so many Americans, we have enjoyed living our lives without giving significant thought to nutrition, exercise, or preventive health. Being Arkansas natives, we both enjoyed a good home-cooked meal of Southern-fried chicken, mashed potatoes with lots of butter, corn, yeast rolls, and of course, strawberry shortcake.

As the years passed by and our children began to adopt the same habits, we found ourselves staring at the scale as it headed in the wrong direction. It all came to pass a few years ago when I (Governor Huckabee) received the wake-up call I needed as my doctors diagnosed me with diabetes. They told me I was digging my grave with a knife and fork, and without a change of lifestyle, I was entering the last decade of my life. I didn't like the sound of that and decided to do something about it. That was 110 pounds ago, and Janet and I have now completed two marathons. We now plan to live to be 100, and are entering the second half of our life.

With the trend of fad diets slowly fading away, we have joined the national fight to help people understand how important it is to achieve good health and to provide the tools with which to do so. Nearly two-thirds of adults—about 65 percent of the population—are overweight or obese. More than 5 percent of adults are morbidly obese. And the numbers continue to get worse. The number of overweight adults is double what it was just 20 years ago, and the morbidly obese are the most rapidly growing subset, having tripled in the last decade.

Today, America's children are heavier than they've ever been. Over 16 percent of kids are overweight, with another 31 percent at risk for obesity. A few years ago, pediatric hospitals had never seen a case of Type 2 diabetes in a preteen. Today, those same hospitals are seeing a dozen cases a week with children as young as eight years old diagnosed with Type 2 diabetes. This may be the first generation whose life expectancy will be shorter than that of their parents.

The impact of being overweight is dramatic, increasing the risk of heart attack, stroke, diabetes, high blood pressure, depression, infertility, reflux disease, high cholesterol and even some types of cancer. The mortality risk for overweight patients is double that of normal-weight individuals.

In addition to the health risks, the cost to society is dramatic. The economic impact of obesity is over $117 billion annually, representing nearly 10 percent of all health-care costs. Generally, health-care costs for an obese individual, are double that of an individual of normal weight.

If you start today, small changes can have big results. Data shows that reducing excess weight by just 10 percent goes a long way toward achieving these goals. Relatively simple and inexpensive strategies to eat healthier and be more active can dramatically improve one's health and well-being, both physically and emotionally.

It's because of this growing epidemic that our family is proud to take part in and actively support Discovery Health Channel's National Body Challenge. Our family is grateful every day that we were able to recognize and correct our bad habits before they overcame our lives. Through a proven program like the National Body Challenge, it is our desire to help other families realize that it's never too late to become healthy.

A healthy lifestyle really does matter!

— **Arkansas Governor Mike Huckabee and First Lady Janet Huckabee**

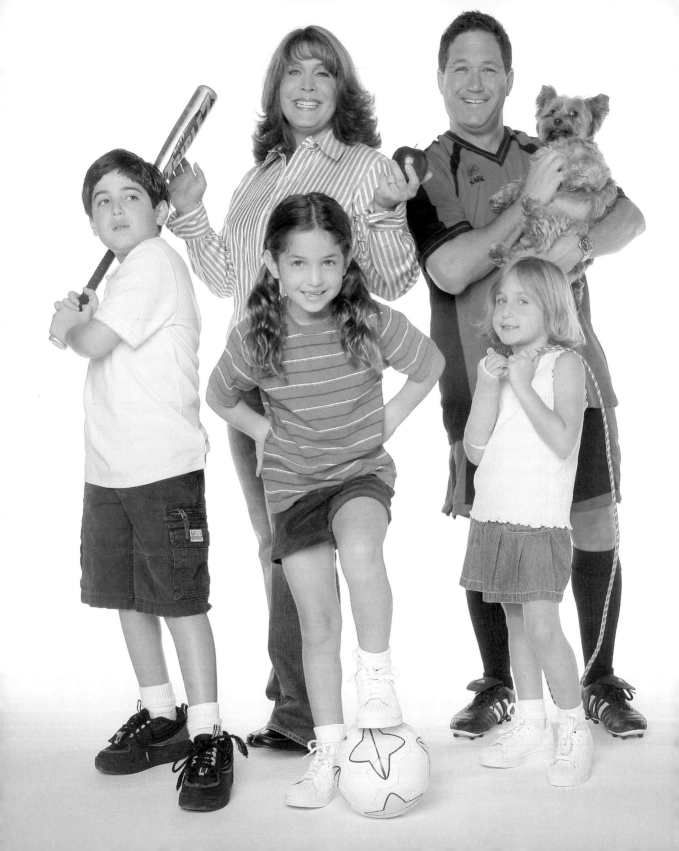

Foreword

By Eileen O'Neill and Dr. John Whyte

Welcome to the National Body Challenge and congratulations for taking this step! Discovery Health Channel created the National Body Challenge as a mechanism to respond to the adult and childhood obesity epidemic that's sweeping the nation. This free, eight-week comprehensive weight-loss and personal-health program provides individuals and families with all the tools and information—on television, online, and through local events—to lead healthier lives.

Log on to **www.discoveryhealth.com** to register for the National Body Challenge, starting December 30, 2005, to take advantage of the amazing information, research, and tools our team has put together to help you with those crucial first steps toward a healthier lifestyle. The challenge runs eight weeks, from January 14 to March 11, 2006. Since its inception in 2004, more than 700,000 people have signed up to take the National Body Challenge. This book highlights the success stories of some of the past participants, and we encourage you to share your story as you take part in the National Body Challenge at **www.discoveryhealth.com**.

Weigh-in online or at one of the six center-court mall events beginning on January 14, 2006. Access the free online diet and fitness resources that provide tools, information, and guidance to lose weight and get fit. Also, tune in to *National Body Challenge: The Family Challenge* on January 15 and 16, 2006, from 8 to 10 P.M. (ET/PT) for more inspiration to stay on track. This two-part special follows the physical and emotional journey of four families as they work together to achieve their personal health goals.

We'd like to thank our partners at the American Heart Association and the American Diabetes Association, as well as the Governor and First Lady of Arkansas, Mike and Janet Huckabee. With partners like these, Discovery Health Channel is able to forge its commitment to producing television that matters for our viewers. And through programs like the National Body Challenge, Discovery Health Channel continues to be a resource you can turn to for further inspiration and information that helps make a positive difference in your life.

— **Eileen O'Neill,** Executive Vice President and
General Manager of Discovery Health Channel; and
Dr. John Whyte, Vice President, Continuing Medical
Education for Discovery Health Channel

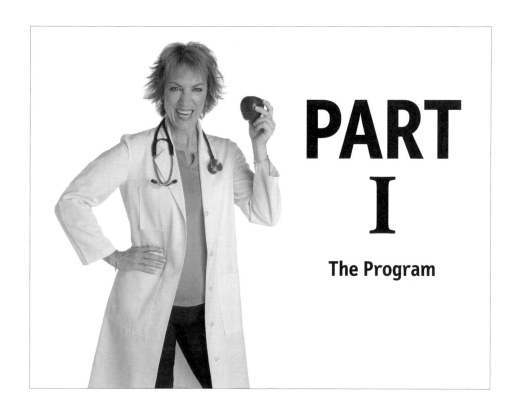

PART
I

The Program

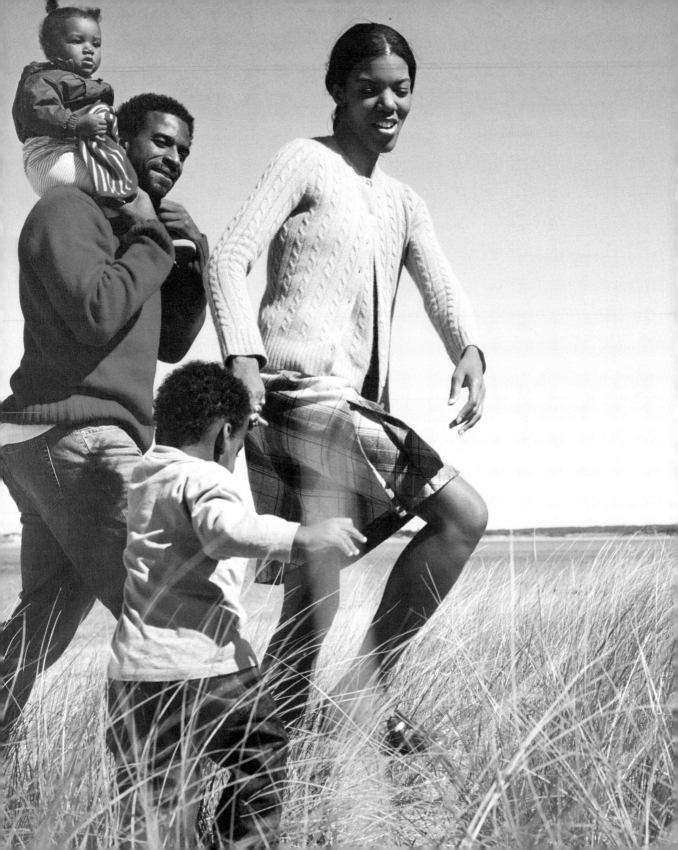

1

Rise *to the* Challenge

This year you're determined to make some changes in your life, starting with your self-care. It's time to wake up and pay attention to your mind and body. Speaking of body, perhaps you've been avoiding stepping on that scale because you suspect that you're heavier than you've ever been. Are those tight waistbands tipping you off to problems with girth control?

And is your expanding waistline impacting your self-esteem and quality of life? Maybe you feel self-conscious about the way you look in your clothes, or perhaps you're just tired of feeling stressed, sluggish, and energy depleted. You'd like to set a good example for your kids, or certain health issues like heart disease and diabetes run in your family and you want to lower your risks for them. Whatever your personal goals, it's time to gain control of your health and—ultimately—your life. Bottom line: You want nothing short of a mental and physical transformation that's sustainable.

Well, congratulations! You've made a smart move in starting the National Body Challenge Success Program for the Whole Family; the first of many smart moves you'll be making in the next eight weeks. Some of you will achieve your goals within this time period, and others will still need to continue to complete their Challenge. That's okay—you can repeat this Challenge as many times as you want. The good news is that however long it takes, you'll get there by staying consistent with the program, and then practicing the basic principles for life.

Through my integrative, holistic Mind, Mouth, and Muscle approach, I'm going to guide you in making stress reduction, proper nutrition, and increased physical activity top priorities. I developed this blueprint for healthy living and have applied it as the program template for the Discovery Health National Body Challenge television series, as well as their Website campaign.

In the 2006 television series, Dr. Lydie Hazan and I worked with four wonderful families in great need of a lifesaving lifestyle makeover. Follow along with the show and this book and you'll learn how to tone your muscles, burn fat, and handle stress and emotions. We'll lay down a foundation that you can build on for the rest of your life. Stick with it and you'll find that you have more energy and improved health. Better yet, the physical changes you experience will manifest other profound changes, such as self-control, confidence, and a healthy self-image. In other words, you'll drop the physical weight of excess fat, and also take a weight off your mind, too. That's the real win/win you're looking to achieve.

I know what you may be thinking right now. You've probably resolved in the past that you'll make positive changes. Then, more often than not, within a few months all those good intentions are circling the drain. You know what to do and you're good at getting started, but you find it hard to stay focused and sustain the effort. Funny how life's stresses emerge and challenge our best intentions, isn't it? Don't worry. We'll teach you how to regroup and learn to navigate those inevitable stress speed bumps, and keep you on track.

Remember, this is all about learning how to become a lifelong winner, not a loser. For instance, how many of you have managed to "lose" some weight only to "find" it again? That's because your goal is not to lose (if you lose your keys, don't you want to find them again?), but to remove excess body fat and keep your muscles in great shape. So don't be part of our national epidemic of losing and finding weight. Instead, concentrate on improving the quality of your mind and body through a healthy lifestyle.

How does this program help you to achieve this goal? Let's count the ways.

First: It Works

The National Body Challenge Success Program for the Whole Family, and the Mind, Mouth, and Muscle formula it's based on, has a track record for being successful when fad diets or trendy exercise programs don't. It's time to get our heads screwed on right and end the confusion around dieting and physical activity. What you'll discover here is based on cutting-edge science. You'll learn about portion control, stress eating, body composition, energy exchange, the importance of Vitamin I = intensity, "toxic fat," how to battle boredom, and learn how to deal with pitfalls and plateaus. I'll also be showing you how not to be a slave to the scale alone. Instead, you'll use your own "clothes-o-meter" belt or pair of jeans that will give you a better idea of the progress you're making as you change your body composition by offloading fat and building muscle. Some of these ideas might be unfamiliar to you, but the proof is in the numbers.

In 2005, hundreds of thousands of people just like you all across the country removed nearly 400,000 pounds of excess weight on the National Body Challenge. That's almost 200 tons and nearly twice the amount that Challengers lost in 2004. That's because each year, participants build upon a body of knowledge and benefit from the experiences of the previous year's Challengers. This puts you in a great position. In this book, you'll find loads of inspiration and information from people who have already been through the program. You only have to read their stories and look at their amazing before-and-after pictures to become charged-up about taking your own transformative mind/body journey.

Second: It's All about You

The National Body Challenge Success Program for the Whole Family can be customized to meet your specific goals and needs whether you're a peri-menopausal woman with an expanding waistline, a stressed-out businessman with high blood pressure, or a shy, chubby ten-year-old. Every member of the family can and should join and do this together. Science shows that the greatest success is achieved when family members work as a team.

This adaptability aspect is important because men and women are hard-wired differently when it comes to how their bodies respond to exercise and fat storage. Women tend to carry more fat than men, and there is a difference in where the fat is deposited. Even among individual men and women, body fat varies dramatically and is dependent upon genetics and lifestyle. Age is a critical factor, too. Every decade, men and women face changes in body composition brought on by hormonal shifts and changes in lifestyle. For example, after age 40, the average woman starts losing muscle, primarily through disuse, as well as the power to burn calories in the same way she did when she was younger. Men lose less than women, but both note significant increases in belly fat as their sex hormones decline.

Then there are the kids. Parents, heads up: The number of overweight and obese children and teens in the U.S. has tripled over the past 40 years. There are 15 million children over age five who are overweight. Researchers predict that this generation of children will be the first to live shorter lives than their parents because of health problems related to their being excessively heavy and sedentary. Teenagers are suffering from health conditions that normally don't occur until mid-life, such as Type 2 diabetes and high blood pressure.

But it's not just about the body. Over 25 percent of kids who report being teased at school about their weight have considered suicide. Depression affects over 30 percent of overweight girls and 20 percent of boys. You moms and dads are your kids' most powerful role models. It is you, through your daily example, who teach children how to live well. Kids can also teach parents a thing or two. Some are learning at school how to eat well and stay active. That's why it's imperative that families work together to prevent or reverse the stressed-out, sedentary lifestyle that leads to obesity and its related medical conditions.

The final way in which this can be personalized is by making it fit your life circumstances. Nobody can be expected to stay on a rigid regimen 100 percent of the time, and I would never ask you to do that. You'll learn about my 80/20 rule (hit your goals 80 percent of the time and leave yourself 20 percent for treats and rest). This is about getting real and learning how to achieve a reasonable and livable balance of healthy lifestyle practices as well as healthy pleasures. Balance is the key. Stick to my 80/20 rule, and as long as you sustain it most of the time, there's wiggle room for those times when life goes awry and those occasions when only a cookie will do.

Third: There's Help Available

This is the only multimedia, integrated health-and-fitness program that provides you with many levels of information and support. Here's how:

- You can watch the National Body Challenge on Discovery Health Channel and follow along as the participants face the same changes and challenges as you do.

- During the National Body Challenge eight-week event, your family can register online at **www.discoveryhealth.com** to take the Challenge. Visit the Website for complete details.

- Registrants 18 years and older who sign on by January 17, 2006 (certain rules and restrictions apply), can get a complimentary trial membership to a health club and free access to Web-based exercises, techniques, and information, so you have no excuses for not working out.

- You can log on to Discovery Health Channel's Website: **www.discovery health.com**, and follow the National Body Challenge week-by-week meal plans, as well as video lectures and tips on eating healthy and getting fit. Also, click on the Website's easy-to-use tools to determine your goals based on your current body composition. Make sure to pay attention to body-fat percentage. One of your goals is to get your body fat into a healthy range. Whatever weight is associated with a healthy percentage of body fat will be your goal weight. Using the Web tools, you'll monitor the calories you eat and those you burn through your more active lifestyle.

- This book will be your guide, providing you with the tools, advice, and encouragement you need to successfully take the National Body Challenge Success Program for the Whole Family and achieve your healthy living goals.

What You Can Expect

First, it's essential to adopt some reasonable expectations. It probably took you a long time to get unfit so be patient as you start the Challenge. The great news is that from the moment you lace up your sneakers and take a walk after eating a healthy meal, you'll be feeling the immediate benefits of more energy and a happier mood as you remove excess body fat and build strong muscles. So, what can you realistically expect? If you start and follow this program consistently, you'll:

- Remove one-half to two pounds of fat per week, with heavier men, women, and kids initially shedding more weight. This will start to slow after you've removed about 70 percent of your body fat.

- Drop water weight of one to five pounds per week over the first several weeks. That's a normal consequence of a reduced intake of sodium and starches that hold body water.

- Build and strengthen muscles that increase your metabolism and your ability to burn calories.

- Increase your strength, endurance, and flexibility so you can enjoy your daily activities more.

- Enhance your enjoyment of life as you share more fun activities with the whole family.

- Manage stress by learning how to regroup when life becomes difficult.

- Eliminate self-destructive habits (smoking, excessive alcohol intake, drug use, stress eating), and substitute them with healthy lifestyle behaviors.

- Sleep more peacefully.

- Decrease the symptoms related to medical conditions you might have, such as arthritis, heart disease, diabetes, menopause, or depression.

- Feel more energized, happier, and hopeful; and less depressed, moody, and anxious.

- Expect to be practicing and honing your healthy lifestyle habits every day of your life. Keep in mind that every step of the journey *is* the journey.

So let's get this Challenge started. Next up, you'll assess where you are now so you can have an accurate record of your progress. Then we'll plunge right into the Mind, Mouth, and Muscle program and take the first steps toward your transformation.

You want to change. Congratulations! Now, let's make it happen.

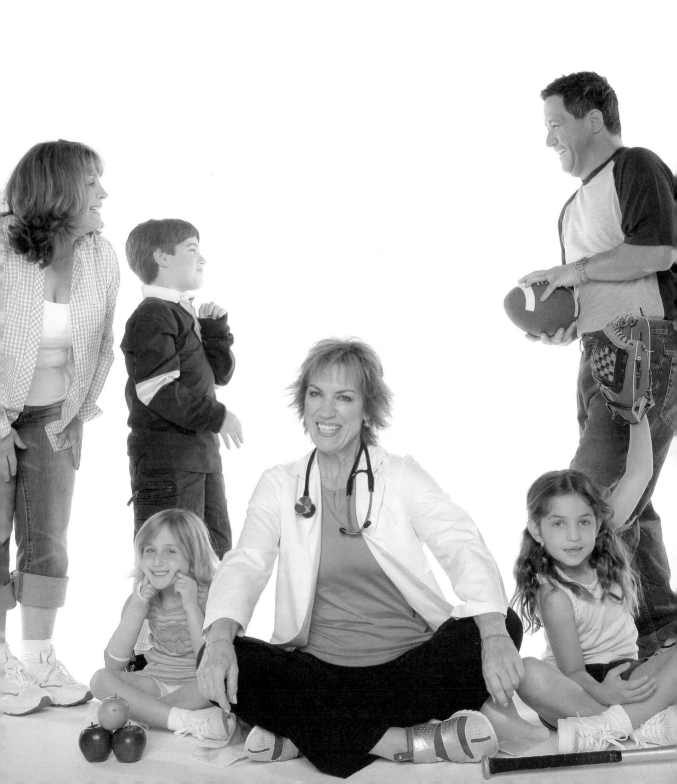

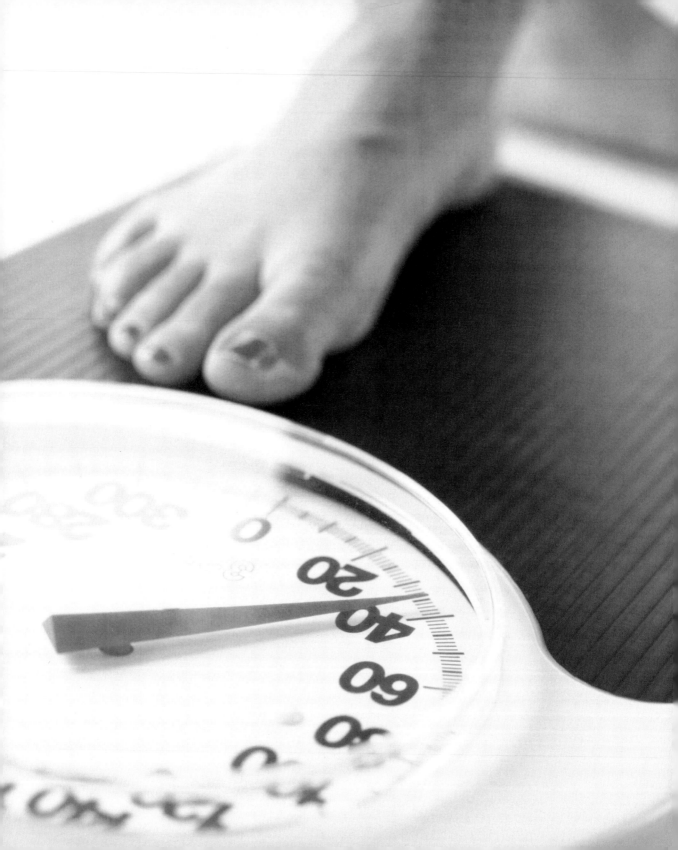

2

Measure Up

Let's get started on your lifetime of healthy living. In my Mind, Mouth, and Muscle template, to ensure lifelong success you must start with your Mind. You need to establish and record your commitment to yourself to work at achieving your healthy lifestyle habits.

I _____,
challenge myself to do my best to eat healthy, whole foods every day, to get up and move around more, to make the time to exercise, and to keep a log of my progress. By doing so, I'm improving the quality of my own life and my loved ones' as well.

_____

Signature

_____

Date

Then, let's see how you measure up by writing down your beginning measurements so you can keep track of them over time. Finally, it's all about lining up the tools and support you'll need to help all members of the family who are taking the Challenge. Here's how to get prepared to be optimally fit:

Take Out a Contract

It's time for everyone in the family to announce their commitment to take the Challenge. Have each person participating sign the National Body Challenge Success Program for the Whole Family Contract. Once it's signed, place it where it can be seen every day—maybe on the refrigerator door or the bathroom mirror. Better still, frame it and hang it up to show your commitment and support for each family member. Sign up, and you're ready to begin!

Why Weight?

What weight are you aiming for? Well, achieving some ideal number on the scale is less important than removing excess body fat, reducing "toxic fat," building muscle mass, and getting healthy.

I wouldn't go so far as to say ditch the scale altogether—record your weight at the beginning, and then check it once a week throughout the Challenge. But this is more about the quality of your body than the quantity. You'll learn more about this in Chapter 3. It is worthwhile, though, to know your body fat percentage, which refers to your amount of body fat in relationship to your total body weight. If you're 150 pounds and 10 percent fat, your body consists of 15 pounds of fat and 135 pounds of lean body mass, which is your bone, muscle, organ tissue, blood, and so on.

You need a certain amount of fat to be healthy. Fat regulates your body temperature, protects your internal organs and tissues, and stores a lot of your body's energy. How much you need is dependent upon whether you're a man or woman, and how old you are.

How do you find out what your body fat percentage is? Well, you can have it analyzed professionally, but these body comp tests can be expensive. However, many gyms have a device to do it for you, and you can buy bathroom

Healthy Range of Body Fat

Age	Females	Males
18–39	21–32 percent	8–19 percent
40–59	23–33 percent	11–21 percent
60–79	24–35 percent	13–24 percent

scales that also measure body fat. Both the devices in the gym and the scales use a very low electrical current to measure body fat.

Knowing your body-fat percentage can help you set realistic weight-removal goals. Remember, weight loss doesn't always mean fat loss. Let's say you're a young woman who currently weighs 130 pounds and you have 23 percent body fat (already in the healthy range). You decide you want to remove 20 pounds. To figure out how many pounds of body fat you have, you'd multiply your weight by your percentage of body fat.

So use this calculation to find out how much fat you have: 130 x .23 = 30. That means you have 30 pounds of fat, and the 100 pounds that's left is lean body mass. Removing 20 pounds of fat would leave you at 110 pounds. But this is neither realistic nor healthy. At 110 pounds, you still need that 100 pounds of lean body mass, so would only have 10 pounds, or 9 percent, body fat. From the chart above, you can see that this is a dangerously low percentage unless you're an elite athlete.

A far better goal is for you to reduce your body fat from 23 percent to 18 percent (in a healthy athletic range). In this case: 130 x .18 = 23 pounds of body fat and 100 pounds of lean body mass. So, to achieve a lean, but healthy 18 percent fat, you would need to remove only 7 pounds of fat, reducing your weight from your current 130 pounds to 123 pounds. Losing more than 7 pounds means that you're losing lean body mass, which is clearly not desirable. So before you decide that you need to "lose weight," remember to consider that "weight" consists of both lean body mass and body fat. Try to keep your weight-loss goals realistic, and remember, keep the calorie-burning muscle and lose only the fat.

You might not have access to having your body fat analyzed, but you can figure out another important figure: your body mass index (BMI). The BMI was established by the federal government as a standard to determine obesity. Your task is to work toward getting it into the healthy range. To find out what your BMI is, use the tool at **http://discovery health.com/tools/calculators/bmi/bmi.html** or the chart on page 14. Find your height in inches in the left-hand column. Look in that column for your weight, and you'll find your BMI in the top column.

Body-Mass Index Chart

BMI	Normal						Overweight					Obese										Extreme Obesity											
	19	20	21	22	23	24	25	26	27	28	29	30	31	32	33	34	35	36	37	38	39	40	41	42	43	44	45	46	47	48	49	50
Height (inches)																Body Weight (pounds)																
58	91	96	100	105	110	115	119	124	129	134	138	143	148	153	158	162	167	172	177	181	186	191	196	201	205	210	215	220	224	229	234	239
59	94	99	104	109	114	119	124	128	133	138	143	148	153	158	163	168	173	178	183	188	193	198	203	208	212	217	222	227	232	237	242	247
60	97	102	107	112	118	123	128	133	138	143	148	153	158	163	168	174	179	184	189	194	199	204	209	215	220	225	230	235	240	245	250	255
61	100	106	111	116	122	127	132	137	143	148	153	158	164	169	174	180	185	190	195	201	206	211	217	222	227	232	238	243	248	254	259	264
62	104	109	115	120	126	131	136	142	147	153	158	164	169	175	180	186	191	196	202	207	213	218	224	229	235	240	246	251	256	262	267	273
63	107	113	118	124	130	135	141	146	152	158	163	169	175	180	186	191	197	203	208	214	220	225	231	237	242	248	254	259	265	270	278	282
64	110	116	122	128	134	140	145	151	157	163	169	174	180	186	192	197	204	209	215	221	227	232	238	244	250	256	262	267	273	279	285	291
65	114	120	126	132	138	144	150	156	162	168	174	180	186	192	198	204	210	216	222	228	234	240	246	252	258	264	270	276	282	288	294	300
66	118	124	130	136	142	148	155	161	167	173	179	186	192	198	204	210	216	223	229	235	241	247	253	260	266	272	278	284	291	297	303	309
67	121	127	134	140	146	153	159	166	172	178	185	191	198	204	211	217	223	230	236	242	249	255	261	268	274	280	287	293	299	306	312	319
68	125	131	138	144	151	158	164	171	177	184	190	197	203	210	216	223	230	236	243	249	256	262	269	276	282	289	295	302	308	315	322	328
69	128	135	142	149	155	162	169	176	182	189	196	203	209	216	223	230	236	243	250	257	263	270	277	284	291	297	304	311	318	324	331	338
70	132	139	146	153	160	167	174	181	188	195	202	209	216	222	229	236	243	250	257	264	271	278	285	292	299	306	313	320	327	334	341	348
71	136	143	150	157	165	172	179	186	193	200	208	215	222	229	236	243	250	257	265	272	279	286	293	301	308	315	322	329	338	343	351	358
72	140	147	154	162	169	177	184	191	199	206	213	221	228	235	242	250	258	265	272	279	287	294	302	309	316	324	331	338	346	353	361	368
73	144	151	159	166	174	182	189	197	204	212	219	227	235	242	250	257	265	272	280	288	295	302	310	318	325	333	340	348	355	363	371	378
74	148	155	163	171	179	186	194	202	210	218	225	233	241	249	256	264	272	280	287	295	303	311	319	326	334	342	350	358	365	373	381	389
75	152	160	168	176	184	192	200	208	216	224	232	240	248	256	264	272	279	287	295	303	311	319	327	335	343	351	359	367	375	383	391	399
76	156	164	172	180	189	197	205	213	221	230	238	246	254	263	271	279	287	295	304	312	320	328	336	344	353	361	369	377	385	394	402	410

According to the National Heart, Lung, and Blood Institute, if you have a BMI of:

- 18.5–24.9, you are at a healthy weight and considered to be at low risk for health problems

- 25–29.9, you're overweight and considered to be at moderate risk

- 30–40, you are obese and considered to be high risk

- Over 40, you are very obese and considered to be at extremely high risk

Those of you in one of the high-risk zones can lower your BMI on the National Body Challenge. Removing even 5 to 10 percent of your body weight can have a significant impact on your health. The amount you need to remove to get your BMI below 25 depends on your height.

Find your height on the chart, and then find the healthy 25 BMI at the top. This will give you a weight to aim for. Subtract it from your current weight to determine how much to remove. For example:

- If you're a 5'5" woman and your BMI is 27, you need to remove 13 pounds to get your BMI below 25; if your BMI is 30, you need to remove 31 pounds to get your BMI below 25.

- If you're a 6' tall man and your BMI is 27, you need to remove 16 pounds to get your BMI below 25; if your BMI is 30, you need to remove 38 pounds to get your BMI below 25.

These are standard guidelines, though, and as with body-fat percentages, may not be valid for everyone. For instance, they do not apply to pregnant women, some elderly people who have lost muscle mass, and those who are more muscular than most of us, such as elite athletes and bodybuilders. If you're not sure whether they apply to you, ask your doctor.

The key for everyone is to combine your body-fat percentage along with your BMI to get the full picture. You want to aim to get both within the healthy ranges for your gender and age. So say you're a 30-year-old woman and you want to get your body-fat percentage between 21 and 32 and your BMI below 25; if you're a 40-year-old man, you want to get your body-fat percentage between 11 and 21 and your BMI below 25. The only way to achieve this is through a fit and healthy lifestyle.

BMI and Kids

These adult guidelines don't apply to children and pre-adolescent teenagers. As children grow, the amount of body fat they have changes, and it differs also in boys and girls. Generally, BMI goes down from chubby babyhood to preschool age and then starts going up again into adulthood. That said, scientists have discovered that a high BMI for their gender, height, age, and weight is a very helpful way of identifying kids and teens that are at risk for becoming significantly overweight adults.

The number of children and teens who are overweight has quadrupled in the last 30 years. The U.S. Department of Health and Human Services wrote a document called *Healthy People 2010,* and in it they noted a goal of reducing overweight children to no more than 5 percent of all kids. Currently, at least 16 percent of all children (and 24 percent of African-American and Hispanic kids) are seriously overweight. This is disturbing because:

- 20–30 percent of overweight kids aged 5 to 11 have high blood pressure, sleep apnea, arthritis, and tend to suffer from depression, anxiety, and social withdrawal.

- 10–50 percent of overweight kids with fatty liver will develop continuing liver inflammation, and finally cirrhosis of the liver as adults.

- 25 percent of the cases of diabetes diagnosed in kids today are Type 2 or related to their being overweight. That's up from 4.5 percent in the early 1990s. It has been predicted that unless things change, one out of every three children born in the year 2000 will have Type 2 diabetes.

- Autopsies done on children and teens showed that there's a strong correlation between BMI and atherosclerotic heart disease. In other words, these kids were already showing signs of heart disease despite their young age.

Is it possible to turn this around? Yes, but only with the whole family *and your doctor* involved.

Regular check-ups so your doctor can weigh and measure your child's growth and development are important, and you have to be assertive about making sure that when your kids visit your health practitioner, their height, weight, and BMI are recorded. You need to know these numbers. A recent study showed that only 75 percent of kids' heights and weights are recorded during regular visits, only 40 percent of the time do health-care providers ask questions about a kid's eating habits and nutrition, and less than 25 percent of the time is children's activity level addressed.

Why is this essential? Because a child's BMI is directly correlated to body fat. You need to know if your child is at risk for becoming overweight or is already overweight enough to necessitate immediate intervention. If doctors can identify these at-risk children early on, they can monitor their body fat, and you can get an early start on helping them prevent adult obesity by making changes in their eating and exercise habits.

For kids, doctors calculate their BMI using a BMI-percentile-for-age calculator adjusted for differences in height, age, and gender. The percentile cut-off points are:

Underweight:	BMI-for-age < 5th percentile
Normal:	BMI-for-age 5th to < 85th percentile
At Risk of Overweight:	BMI-for-age 85th to < 95th percentile
Overweight:	BMI-for-age > 95th percentile

So your doctor will correlate age, gender, and BMI to be able to determine if your child is at the 85–94 percentile of BMI for age and thus at risk for becoming overweight, or is over 95 percent and already overweight. Be your child's advocate and ask that the doctor provide this information. With numbers in hand, you can implement the changes you need to make to help your child achieve the healthiest weight and body composition he or she deserves and avoid the high cholesterol, the Metabolic Syndrome, fatty liver, Type 2 diabetes, and high blood pressure that pediatricians are noting in epidemic numbers around the U.S.

So be alert and make sure you're getting the real lowdown during your child's physical exam and laboratory reports so that you can make goals and achieve them optimally.

You'll find the growth charts consisting of percentile curves showing the distribution of body measurements that pediatricians use at **www.cdc.gov/growthcharts** so you can plot your kids' progress yourself.

Exercise Some Girth Control

Your waist measurement is a particularly important number when it comes to your health. To find yours, use a cloth tape measure around the smallest part of your waist across the belly button (don't pull the tape too tight). The goal for women is to get below 35 inches; for men, it's to get below 40 inches. This is because where you carry your weight is even more important than how much you carry. If you have excess body fat inside your abdomen, giving you that apple-shaped body, it's a pretty good indication that you have excess inner abdominal fat—what I call "toxic fat" deep in your belly surrounding your liver and other organs.

Too much of this fat puts you at greater risk for heart disease, high blood pressure, diabetes, and certain types of cancer. In fact, a study at the University of Texas Southwestern confirms that people with large waists and thin thighs have an even higher cardiovascular-disease risk than people who have more fat but store their weight in their lower bodies.

Also, take that tape measure to your chest, hips, and thighs. That's more for aesthetic reasons but heck, that's important, too. If you look good, you feel good. You'll be keeping these measurements every week on the Challenge to chart how you're really doing.

Use a "Clothes-O-Meter"

On the National Body Challenge, you're going to be changing your body composition, removing fat, and building muscle. As you now know, muscle weighs more than fat, so you might see your first changes in the size of your body rather than in numbers on the scale. You'll likely get a better idea of your progress by using what I call a "clothes-o-meter." For guys it might be a "belt-o-meter" that right now doesn't quite buckle around your waist. For women it might be a "jeans-o-meter" or some other tight piece of clothing that you can get on but can't fully button or zip up. Your goal is to fit into it.

Try it on once a week before you step onto your scale or body-fat analyzer. As your size changes and your "clothes-o-meter" finally fits, choose a tighter one until you finally arrive at your goal. Then, you'll be wearing your "clothes-o-meter" all the time, since it's the size you always aimed for and finally achieved.

To maintain your focus and motivation, hang your "clothes-o-meter" somewhere in full sight in your closet so it will be a daily reminder.

Chart Your Starting Stats

In the best of all worlds, I'd recommend that each family member have a physical exam and also have a baseline amount of laboratory testing done before starting the Challenge. Most health departments, schools, your doctor's office, or health clinics can easily obtain accurate height, weight, and blood pressure, as well as tape measurements. Some will also conduct simple cholesterol and glucose tests. Just start the Challenge and keep track of your weight, body fat, size, and tape measurements. Make a copy of this chart for each member of the family taking the Challenge.

Name _____

Measurements

Height _____

Weight _____

Waist Measurement Across Your Belly Button
(adults only) _____
Desirable: less than 35" for women or 40" for men

Clothing Size
(men belts; women jeans; children pants or dress) _____

Body-Mass Index (BMI) _____
For desirable ranges see page 14

Body-Fat Percentage _____
For desirable ranges, see page 13

Optional Medical Evaluations

Blood Pressure _____
Desirable: up to 120/80
High: 140–159/90 99
Very high: 160/100 and up

Total Cholesterol _____
Desirable: less than 200 mg/dl (adults); less than 170 mg/dl (ages 2–19)
Borderline: 200–239 mg/dl (adults); 170–199 mg/dl (ages 2–19)
High-risk: 240 and over mg/dl (adults); 200 and over mg/dl (ages 2–19)

HDL _____
Desirable: above 40 (adults and children)

LDL _____

Desirable: less than 100 (adults and children)
Acceptable: 100–129 (adults); less than 110 (ages 2–19)
Borderline high: 130–159 (adults); 110–129 (ages 2–19)
High: 160 and up (adults); 130 and up (ages 2–19)

Triglycerides _____

Normal: less than 150
Borderline high: 150–199
High: 200–499
Very high: 500 and up

Blood Glucose _____

Desirable: less than 120

Thyroid Profile _____

(if your doctor feels it's necessary by history and physical exam)

Liver Enzymes _____

(to rule out fatty liver infiltration)

Photograph the Evidence

You only have to look at our dramatic before-and-after photographs of people who have already taken the Challenge to realize the impact of them. Wouldn't you like to have your own record of your progress? Take a full-figure before picture in a bathing suit or workout clothes at the start, and another at the end of this Challenge. Or perhaps you want to take photos in your "clothes-o-meter" before and after the Challenge.

Write It Off

Research has shown that those who keep track of their progress do the best. That means just simply writing down how you're doing with motivation, focus, and stress (Mind), eating (Mouth), and physical activity (Muscle).

On separate pages of your journal, write down three to five goals in each category. Then keep track of each goal as you participate in the Challenge.

Under Mind, you might want to manage stress better, control your anger, and be more patient with your spouse and kids. Go into detail. When it comes to handling stress, it could be that you need to learn how to be more assertive and establish reasonable boundaries with your employer so that you're no longer working pressure-filled 12-hour days. You could decide to stop and listen to your children when they're trying to talk to you instead of being distracted by chores.

On the Mouth page, you might write about controlling your stress overeating, especially during those times of day you ritually stuff yourself: after 3 P.M. or between dinner and bedtime when you're crashed in front of the television. Maybe you want to start eating a healthy breakfast in the morning rather than polishing off the kids' leftovers or stopping at your local java joint on the way to work for that 16-ounce, 320-calorie vanilla latte and 380-calorie blueberry muffin that also has 28 grams of sugar. Perhaps you want to start having healthy, well-balanced family dinners around the table with the TV off.

Muscle is all about simply being more active. How about buying a pedometer (to count your steps) and wearing it on your waistband to calculate just how much you get up and move? Make a specific plan to walk more until you eventually reach about 10,000 steps every day. Start cross-training by adding yoga, Pilates, tai chi, or new cardio equipment into your workouts. Do more outdoor activities as a family: Learn to roller skate, ride bikes, or go for hikes together. Heck, just move more! Remember, you won't *remove* weight unless you *move* weight!

Now, the key is to stay on top of this by keeping track. No matter what, commit to writing something every day; just a little update in each of your Mind, Mouth, and Muscle categories. It's like talking to yourself. Kids should use the same Mind, Mouth, and Muscle journal, but a parent must sign off on the journal each day. That means that the child is accountable, and the parent is monitoring each child's progress.

As an example of journaling, here are some excerpts from the journal of Karen Staitman, 41, of Westlake Village, California (read more about her on page 195), who was a great success story during the 2004 National Body Challenge.

> My biggest challenge was getting started. I'm taking care of a family and two businesses, which usually leaves no time for me except for a shower in the morning. My husband is so supportive and is helping me out even more than he usually does. He too is very busy, so we've had to juggle the responsibilities between us.
> It was all so exciting and new just a couple of weeks ago. And to top it all off, I'm dropping weight, which of course you would think would motivate me

even more. But getting up Monday morning at 5:00 was really difficult. Get-
ting up Tuesday and Wednesday was even harder.

My biggest success this week was fitting into an old pair of jeans. I keep
several old pairs in my closet, mostly because I refuse to buy new ones at a
larger size. I've shed some weight, and I feel compelled to try on a pair. First I
put my left leg in followed by my right. Then I slowly wriggled them around my
tush and lay down on the bed to zip them up. You won't catch me out in public
with them on, but as I look at myself in the mirror I'm smiling anyway because
I'm a pant leg closer than I was last week to reaching my goal!

Revisit your journal week after week to look at your progress and your challenges. Your writings will help when you hit those pitfalls and plateaus and you need a little motivation and encouragement. Leaf through your journal and see what progress you've made. You are your own best cheerleader, after all. And you are your child's greatest teacher and supporter. If you both do well, it's a terrific win/win.

As well as keeping a journal, it's a good idea to keep daily food and exercise logs for each member of the family. Why bother? After all, don't you know what you're putting in your mouth and whether or not you've exercised? Well, your logs will help you stay on top of things and make you accountable: Did you eat breakfast every day this week, did you have six small meals every day, and did you drink enough water? It will keep you honest, also, when you have to put those check marks next to your cardio and strength-training workouts.

There's another really good reason to log your food intake and activity: It will help you be more successful in removing weight. The National Weight Control Registry, which monitors people who have removed at least 30 pounds and kept it off for a year, has reported that a majority of its 3,500 participants who have removed an average of 66 pounds and kept it off for five years monitor their progress by keeping food journals. Other studies have shown similar results. The lesson here? Write it down, write it off!

Find food and exercise logs that you can copy and use daily on pages 25 and 27. You'll also find logs online at Discovery Health Channel's Website: **www.discoveryhealth.com** and click on National Body Challenge.

So that you know exactly what we're talking about, we've included a sample filled-in daily food log and a week's worth of daily exercise logs.

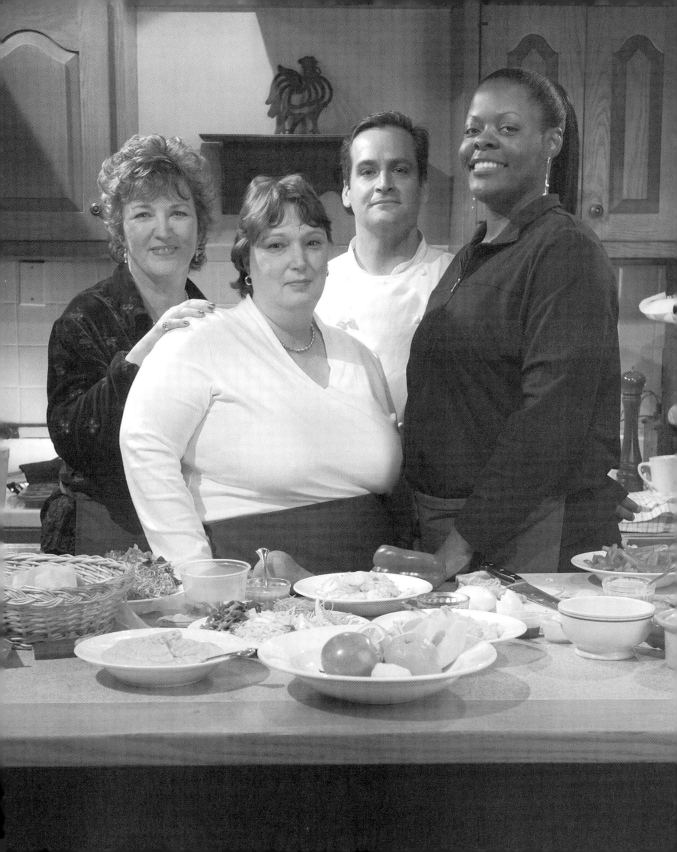

SAMPLE FOOD LOG

S	M	T	W	T	F	S	DAY #	DATE

FOOD

Time	Item	Cal.	Reason
7 am	wheat toast (1 piece)	150	hungry
	2 scrambled eggs	198	
	tomato juice	41	
10:30	apple, 1 oz. cheese	181	hungry
1:00	green salad w/chicken	198	hungry
	pretzels	110	
3:30	15 almonds	104	bored
	celery w/ light cream cheese	84	
6:15	salmon, creamed spinach		hungry
	& red potatoes	260	
8:00	sugar-free popsicle	25	craving
8:00			

Total Cal.	1351

WATER

FOOD LOG

S M T W T F S	DAY #	DATE

FOOD

Time	Item	Cal.	Reason

	Total Cal.	

WATER

SAMPLE EXERCISE LOG

S M T W T F S	DAY #	DATE

CARDIO

Type	Minutes
Running	45
Swiming	30
WALKING **NUMBER OF STEPS**	9012

STRENGTH TRAINING

Type	Weight/Reps
Crunches	50
Lunges	50
Bench press	10/15
Leg press	100/12

FLEXIBILITY

Type	Minutes
Yoga class	45
Stretching	15

Generally, you will not be performing all three types of activity in one day. You are encouraged to alternate exercises. The above provides only an example for filling in the log.

EXERCISE LOG

S M T W T F S	DAY #	DATE

CARDIO

Type	Minutes
WALKING **NUMBER OF STEPS**	

STRENGTH TRAINING

Type	Weight/Reps

FLEXIBILITY

Type	Minutes

De-Junk Your Kitchen

To give yourself a fighting chance of staying the course, clean out the fridge and cupboards. Get rid of foods containing refined processed sugars and high fat. Stock up on smart, whole foods including fruits and vegetables in a variety of colors; and whole grains including multigrain cereals and breads, brown rice, barley, and whole-wheat pasta.

Schedule a regular time to grocery shop, and go armed with a shopping list.

De-Clutter Your Environment

You can't take that walk if you can't find your sneakers. Patiently begin the task of tidying up critical areas of your house. These are the places you'll need to access to eat, sleep, chill out, work, and exercise in. Organize your kitchen cabinets. You can't cook healthfully if you can't locate ingredients, pots, and pans.

Do the same in your bedroom closet. Just where are those sneakers? How about your workout clothing? Can you find your athletic socks and your gym bag? You can't exercise if you can't find the equipment. Get organized so that the room you work out in is easy to access, the equipment is in working order, and the TV or radio is in there to keep you going. If you have a personal music player, program it with your favorite upbeat songs to get you motivated to move.

Here's a radical thought: Get the family involved in cleaning up their rooms, closets, and the garage instead of wasting time on the couch in front of the TV overeating. Reward everyone who does well with something that doesn't involve food, like a special toy for the kids, or shopping for the teens. This is where family efforts can really pay off.

Work Out an Exercise Plan

Get the right clothing and shoes. You'll need comfortable shirts, shorts, and sweats that allow you to move freely. Go to an athletic apparel store and get fitted with appropriate shoes. The best are cushioned cross-trainers that are wide enough to support you as you exercise. Wear socks specifically made for exercising for greater comfort and to banish blisters.

If you've registered with the National Body Challenge, take advantage of your Bally's Total Fitness free trial membership available if you register by January 17, 2006 (certain rules and restrictions apply; go online to **discoveryhealth.com** for more details). Experiment and try out gym classes, group training, or just walking, hiking, or biking with a friend. Or if that walk is a special time to just enjoy the quiet and regroup, then go solo. Schedule your exercise just as you would any other appointment. Put your exercise gear out so you're always ready to get active: in the car, near the treadmill, or by the front door.

Enlist Support

You can't make major lifestyle changes by yourself: You need a support system. Support from your partner is especially important. So make the National Body Challenge a true family affair. Get your spouse and kids involved and you'll all end up healthier for it. Hey, don't forget your pet. There's nothing like unconditional love to help you along with your Challenge. Walk your dog and you'll both get fit: another win/win situation!

Do the National Body Challenge with a friend or group of friends. Enlist your extended family, your workmates, heck, even your book club. Having a workout buddy and someone to call or e-mail when you're experiencing a particularly tough day can be motivating. The three Challengers who participated in the 2005 televised Challenge: Laura Armstrong, Beth Powell, and Brian Ross, all found this to be true.

"Being on a team where there were other people like me and we plowed through this together was a thrill and a half," says Laura. "That was really what I needed. If I hadn't had that kind of support, I wouldn't have been as successful as I was." (To see just how successful she and the others were, see page 179.)

"We adored each other and still keep in touch," says Beth, "and I think that was key to the success of it: We were all pulling for each other."

For Brian, accountability to his teammates was a big factor, too. Friends, neighbors, and work colleagues can also be cheerleaders and motivators. "My friends would write e-mails saying you look great, keep it up, good work," says Brian. "Everyone was so into it."

You'll also get plenty of support from the National Body Challenge community online at: **www.discoveryhealth.com**.

Tips and Tools

Before you get started, make yourself familiar with the National Body Challenge Web pages at **www.discoveryhealth.com**.

Now that you're all set to go, let's learn more about the Mind, Mouth, and Muscle approach.

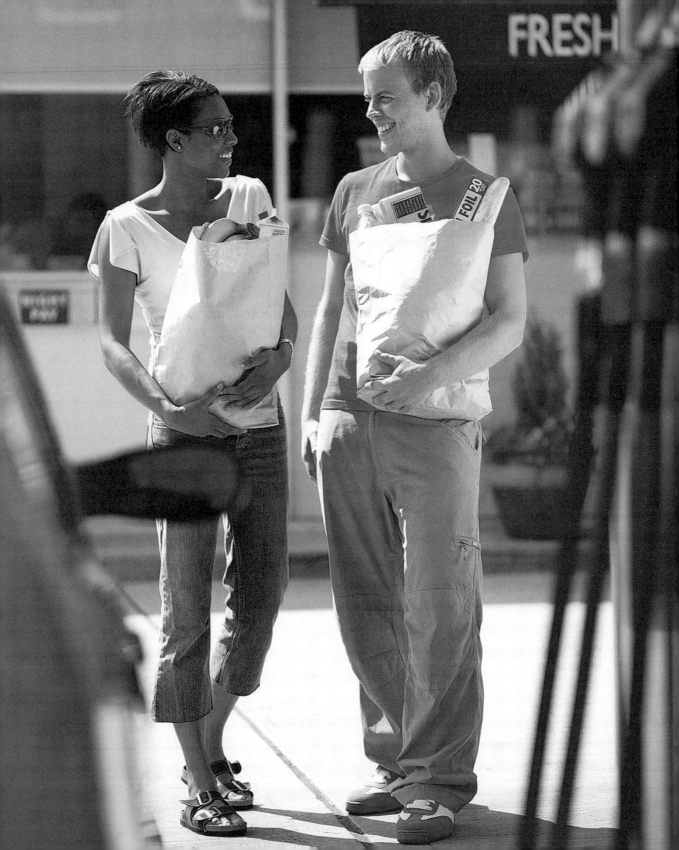

3

The
Mind, Mouth,
and Muscle
Formula

You've come to the National Body Challenge Success Program for the Whole Family looking for a way to finally achieve transformation and to sustain that change for life. I've based the program on my own approach, which is supported by the best clinical information out there. I call it the Mind, Mouth, and Muscle Plan. It's about showing how your mind affects your body.

If you connect the dots, your focus and attitude determines how and what you eat and exercise. In other words, you're getting a blueprint for healthy living, a total mental and physical fitness program. This program is successful because it's holistic, it's integrative, it's family oriented, it's intergenerational, and you'll have the ability to maintain it for the long haul. Better yet, it's cheat-proof! You'll find no fad diets here, just sound data based on the most recent breakthroughs in science.

Fat, and Where It's At

One of the important aspects of this approach, and what makes it so different from other programs, is that it has to do with the issue of fat versus body composition. We're talking about the quality of your body, not the quantity of it. Fat is important, but it's only one data byte. You can be an average weight for your height, age, and gender, but be unhealthy because your body composition isn't good. You can't be optimally healthy if you look at the numbers on the scale and miss the fact that your body fat is way too high.

I saw a woman one day who was 38 years old, 5'4", and 115 pounds. She thought she was healthy because her scale weight was "normal," but was puzzled as to why she felt so drained of energy all the time. I said, "Why don't you step on the body composition analyzer and let me see what your body composition looks like?" We came to find out that her body fat was high at 33 percent instead of the 20 to 25 percent it should have been. I knew right away that in order to achieve her scale weight, she must have been starving herself and simply didn't have energy to exercise.

She looked embarrassed, and admitted that she didn't eat very much because she wanted to keep that size-6 body. I explained to her that it's not about body weight; it's about achieving a healthy balance of fat and muscle. She had lost a lot of muscle by not eating. Lots of women chronically undereat, interspersing the starving with bingeing. This plays havoc with your body composition, leaving you with less muscle and more fat in the end.

Ironically, though, you can end up in the normal weight zone. When you eat smart and exercise, you build muscle and preserve bone and can end up weighing more but being more compact, with sexy curves, and a smaller size because fat occupies more space and muscle weighs more. Remember, when you try to zip up your pants in the morning, that isn't muscle getting in the way!

Contrast this woman with another patient. She was roughly the same height and age but weighed 140 pounds with 22 percent body fat. She'd recently removed over 40 pounds through healthy nutrition and exercise. She'd minimized her body fat and maximized her muscle tone. More fit, she wears the same size as her starving counterpart. In the end, who's healthier? Woman number two. Why? Because too much body fat can increase your risk of breast cancer. But this doesn't just apply to women; men put themselves at increased risk for prostate cancer.

It's also very important to know not just how fat you are, but where the fat is. Both women and men need to be especially concerned if they have too much fat in the belly area. In other words, if you're a woman and your waist is bigger than 35 inches, or if you're a man and your waist is above 40 inches, you have too much belly fat. (You can also get a clue if your waist size is bigger than your hips or you start looking like an apple.) This indicates that you have what's called visceral fat coating your internal organs, especially the liver.

Even if you're average weight but too much of your fat is distributed inside the belly, then you're at risk for the *metabolic syndrome.* This is defined as having too much of this visceral fat combined with other factors such as low levels of HDL ("good") cholesterol, high blood pressure, and insulin resistance (leading to abnormal blood sugar levels). People with the metabolic syndrome are at increased risk for coronary heart disease, stroke, and Type 2 diabetes. For that matter, the association between excessive inner abdominal obesity and diabetes is so strong that experts now refer to this relationship as "diabesity." According to the American Heart Association, 20 to 25 percent of American adults have it.

Although it was once most common in middle-aged adults, an increasing number of children and teens are now being diagnosed with the metabolic syndrome. Here's a statistic that should give us pause: U.S. teenagers are the most overweight of any in industrialized countries. Plus, there's alarming new data showing that overweight teenagers who are exposed to secondhand cigarette smoke have five times more risk of developing metabolic syndrome, and those who smoke are six times more likely to get it. And what's really of concern is that obese kids and teens who have the metabolic syndrome will have a poor quality of life due to the medical conditions, and a shorter life at that. So come on—let's nip it in the bud right now.

Hopefully, I've convinced you that it's really all about body composition, not scale weight. You can see how important it is to look at body-fat percentage and amount, and optimize your health by trying to keep it to a minimum. But how?

The Cheat-Proof Program

Now here's why this program is a wonderful, fabulous, new way of going about it: You cannot optimize body fat by cheating. I could tell you to reach a certain weight, and you could hit it by starving on your own and think you were so healthy, when in fact, you've likely lost muscle tissue along with the fat. Well, here's the beauty of it: If I tell you to achieve a specific body fat, it's impossible to cheat, because the only way to achieve that is through appropriate nutrition and fitness.

This quality versus quantity issue also means that you'll be at a smaller clothing size at a higher weight than you'd anticipated. Why? Because we know for a fact that muscle weighs more than fat. There's something else very interesting. A pound of fat is anywhere from three to four times the size of a pound of muscle. It's very important to understand that you can actually be a certain size but your weight is way off from what you think it should be because you have more heavy muscle than you had before, and therefore it's affecting your scale numbers. And that's true for males and females.

Take a Load Off

To remove physical weight, it's important that you remove mental weight. What is mental weight? For women it could be anything from getting stuck in the "rumination rut" to perfectionism. Stress overeating is another chunk of weight for them. Men stress over providing for their families. Often, their work is so much more important to them than working out. They just can't make it to a fitness facility to whack out stress in the morning before going to a board meeting.

So you see that those aren't just fat pounds on you. They're stress pounds, pain pounds, and frustration pounds. I've found that for most people, so much of their excess weight is a reflection of what's going on in their lives. Once you achieve better balance and establish a healthy lifestyle, funny how you tend to shed the body fat.

Kids aren't immune. Work done at the Children's National Medical Center in Washington, D.C., has shown that kids with a higher BMI are dissatisfied with their body image and have lower self-esteem than their slimmer peers. Tell me that isn't stressful. Children take their cues from their parents. Please remember this: If you signed on to have a child, you also signed on to be a teacher. And if you think your children aren't watching you while you stuff down a bag of nasty stuff when you're pressured, think back to your own childhood for just one second and recall your own parents' attitude toward food. What do you remember from them?

I remember that my mother ate healthfully for most of her life, but she was also someone who was blessed with "happy genes." She routinely ate chocolate—never large amounts, only treats here and there—but it worked for her. And she's 90 years old now, and not dependent on anything other than arthritis medicine. My father ate lots and lots of protein but not enough vegetables, and I remember him working very hard. But I also remember his heart attack at the age of 63 and his coronary bypass, because I was a physician working with his medical team. So I connected my own dots.

How about you connecting your dots? Here's what I want you to do. Like the families on the show, draw your family tree. Put down grandparents, mom and dad, brothers, and sisters, and write down who was overweight. That means if they were anywhere from 20 to about 30 pounds overweight, mark them "overweight." Also record those relatives who are or were at least 40 pounds overweight. Above their name, I want you to write down "obese." Now look at your own children: Do you see a pattern? It's very eye-opening, isn't it? If two parents are obese, the chance of a child becoming obese is 60 to 80 percent. If both parents are lean, the chance drops to 9 percent. Do not, though, use genetics as an excuse. People with a strong genetic tendency toward overweight or obesity come by it honestly. It's not their fault, but it is their responsibility to optimize every chance to fight it.

Fifty percent of overweight children and teens will become overweight and obese adults. But another 50 percent will not. That's due to lifestyle and environment. If parents become proactive and change, it makes it more possible for kids and teens to do the same, thus avoiding obesity and its health-related conditions. *Genetics may load the gun, but environment pulls the trigger.* So if you have challenging genetics, you want to minimize problems by creating a productive environment; you'll learn how to do that in this book and by watching the show. If you have great genetics, you should optimize that magnificent advantage. You'll do that by getting out there and moving.

Now that you've done the family tree, here's another exercise: Sit down and write down your own entire weight history from birth until now. If you can't remember weight, make it clothing size. Just for grins, pull out a family photo album. How many of you would give your right arm to look like you did at 20? Oh, and by the way, at 20 you were complaining about your weight! What's that all about? Look at yourself over time and connect the dots. Now connect your weight to stressful events in your life. If there was a time you were overweight, what was your stress level? Did you become a stress overeater? Or if you were thin, were you a stress undereater? It could go either way depending on how severe the stress was. Toxic stress, the kind that can drag on and leave you besieged, beat up, and aged before your time tends to increase your appetite for comfort food and pack on that visceral fat.

Also, look at any times that you were paying more attention to exercise and healthy eating. Remember what you did and how you felt? How you were eating then? Pull out those pictures from your album, close your eyes, and recall how great you felt. We're going to be using that same formula.

That brings us to the technical side of things: how you eat and how you move your body. I'm giving you a template for healthy living, but customize it for yourself. Feel free to get on out there and belly up to that buffet table of options in this program. You have this choice when you get dressed in the morning. If you're a woman, don't you do this when you're figuring out what kind of makeup works for you? You don't just use one kind. No, it takes experimentation.

I'll bet you've had some interesting experiences with bad hair days and bad hairdressers, haven't you? If you're a guy, then recall how long it took you to figure out which suits and colors worked for you. By trial and error, you finally got a system that worked. Bottom line: It's how you learn. So here's what you're going to do: Play around. Be adventuresome. Remember my favorite quote from Helen Keller: "Life is either a daring adventure or nothing at all."

So get on out there, and if you fall down on your little feminine or masculine behind and make a mistake, then get up, get out there, and learn some more. Show your kids it's okay to make mistakes, because that's the way you eventually learn how to live well.

Men, Women, and Children

Speaking of feminine and masculine, we've learned from science that so much of this fitness issue is gender specific. We now have the Office of Research on Women's Health at the National Institutes of Health. Through them we're learning about the differences between males and females. The Institute of Medicine published a manual called *Does Sex Matter?* approximately four or five years ago. In it, scientists first began to seriously consider differences between men and women.

Guys, you do have an advantage over us women even if you're a train wreck! You have more androgens on board: Those are male sex hormones that allow you to be able to maintain your muscle mass as you age. Consequently, you're able to maintain a better metabolic edge over women, build muscle faster, and yes indeed, drop weight faster. This is a tough reality for women, so your job is to encourage the women in your life, and don't compare your success to theirs, since women will always remove fat slower than men.

Women also have other gender-specific medical concerns that directly impact upon their metabolism. Metabolism is affected by three factors: genetics, thyroid function, and muscle mass. You'll be hearing more about how to optimize your muscles later. But, women should pay special attention to monitoring their thyroid function because many walk around unaware that they have hypothyroidism. A simple blood test is necessary to confirm the diagnosis.

Ladies, do not compare yourself to your husband, your father, your son, or any male in your life. You're apples and oranges. Yes, you're both fruit, but you're apples and oranges. Compete with yourself on this one.

Age is a factor, too, as we're learning from the National Institute on Aging. So listen up, baby boomers: If you're in your 40s, 50s, and early 60s, there's no question that your metabolism is starting to slow down a little bit, partially due to reduced physical activity. But there's also another thing that takes place: Your sex hormones are declining, and this absolutely has an effect on metabolic function. We believe it may have an impact on the ability of fat cells to efficiently release the fat in them.

So here's where you really want to pay attention. All through your life, and especially after the age of 40, it's exceptionally important to remember the Energy Balance Equation: What goes in must come out. That means you must be more mindful of the quality and quantity of your foods and the amount of physical activity you need to work them off. Don't fall asleep at the meal and end up wearing your extra calories. Also, after 40, it's really important to add more of what I call "Vitamin I," or intensity, to your physical activity.

In regard to children, a lot of the same gender issues apply, especially as they're entering their adolescent and teen years. There's no question that teenage girls start to pick up more fat as they begin their menstrual cycles. Current statistics show that while teenage boys either maintain or somewhat increase their physical activity, teenage girls' activity levels plummet as they prefer to spend time on the phone or in front of the television. It certainly doesn't help that most high schools have eliminated a large percentage of their physical-education programs, leaving teens with no incentive to work out at all. Again, we destroy our own metabolic edge.

For different reasons and in different ways, all of us—men, women and children—need to boost our metabolism by keeping our muscles in good shape. Starting to get more active is like building a fire, and then you need to stoke that fire throughout your life. It's your metabolic fire, and it will serve you well by being a calorie-burning furnace. It's very important to understand that every pound of active muscle on our body burns between 35 to 50 calories per day to maintain itself. Fat, on the other hand, only requires anywhere from 5 to 10 calories. So I'd rather go for the muscle: Give me that big Humvee engine instead of that little moped engine that's not burning calories efficiently.

So let's go ahead and take a closer look at each of the Mind, Mouth, and Muscle parts of the program. As you begin, please realize that most people look at these three elements and find that there's one in particular that's a real challenge. Maybe you eat well but have an "antibody" response to exercise and break out into a cold sweat when you think about it. Or perhaps you're a man, woman, or kid who just loves to get out there and exercise, but you eat enough for a small country! And how about you folks who have mastered the nutrition and physical-activity elements, but are stressed out of your minds most of the time?

The bottom line is that you will practice the Mind, Mouth, and Muscle principles until you achieve a balance that works for you. The rule is that to achieve optimal mental and physical fitness, you have to honor all three elements. You'll fail if you try to ignore one. So be patient. I'm going to show you how to achieve that balance.

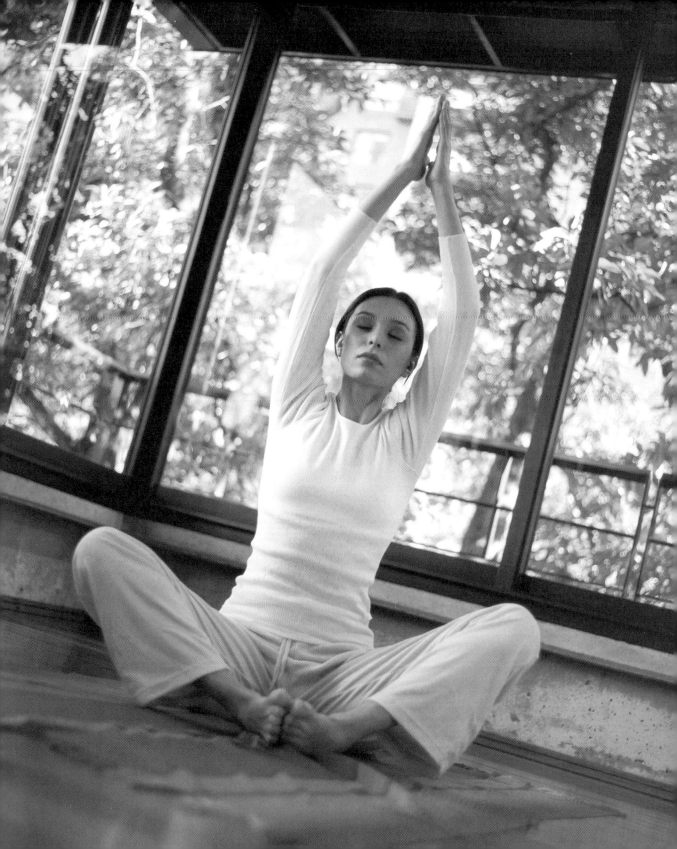

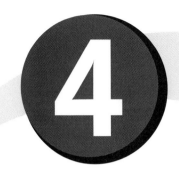

Mind

The mind is an absolutely crucial element to your success. Your mind is where you harbor your focus and motivation, the driving forces to get you started and keep you going for life. You'll notice that I put it before mouth and muscle. Why did I do that?

Well, simply because without your head screwed on right, this whole thing isn't going to work. Look, it's not rocket science to learn how to eat well and move more. The hardest part is keeping on track mentally. Here are some ways to do that.

Take Aim

By rising to this challenge, you've gone from contemplation to action. You're ready now to make some changes. But why are you so ready right now? And is the reason for your need to change powerful enough to sustain you through life's stresses and tough times?

Here's an exercise that I want you to do: Get comfortable somewhere with your journal and write down your motivations for doing this Challenge. Start by asking yourself, "Why am I interested in making changes?" Now make a laundry list—it can be as long as you like—of all the reasons you can think of. There are no right or wrong items to write down. This is your personal inventory, and anything goes.

Some of the things that I hear all the time in my practice are: I want to prevent myself from getting a medical condition that runs in my family, I already have heart disease or diabetes and I want to reverse it, I'm self-conscious about my appearance, I'm lacking energy, my closet looks like a department store with ten sizes hanging in it depending on where I land on the scale, and I wear "hide-it" clothes all the time. Maybe *belt* is a four-letter word to you, or elastic has become your best friend?

When you've finished your list, read through it and answer this question: Would you consider all these to be powerful reasons? I'll bet you said yes, didn't you? But if they are that powerful, you'd think you would have made the change before now. Isn't that interesting? It's because these are what I call "global" motivations. These are general reasons for wanting to transform your life, and they're a great starting point. The problem, though, is that often they do not exert a wrenching enough pull on you when you're tired, stressed, hankering for comfort food, and looking for an excuse to plunk down in front of the TV with a bag of chips instead of lacing up your sneakers and going for a walk. Yes, you'd like to fit into smaller-size jeans, but in the moment, you want the chips more.

Global motivations tend to erode as the day wears on and you wear out. They're just too general, and most of the time they're not specific enough to stop you in your self-destructive tracks. Honestly, who cares about preventing heart disease when, by 5 P.M., most men and women are in a serious state of overwhelm and can't remember their names let alone the good intentions they had that morning. This is when you need to pull out the big guns: your "target" motivations. Think of your global motivations as the outer rings of an archery target. Your target motivations are the bull's-eye, and that's what we need to reach. See the diagram on the next page.

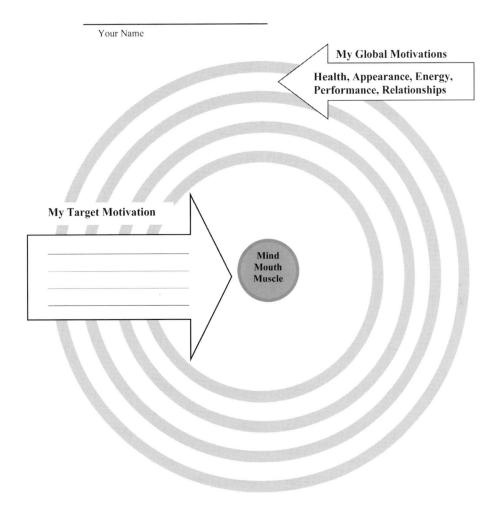

Your Name

My Global Motivations

Health, Appearance, Energy, Performance, Relationships

My Target Motivation

Mind
Mouth
Muscle

Target motivations are the real deal. They are why you're actually doing this Challenge; and most people have to dig deep, past the global motivations, to find them. The target motivation is what you think about every time you have a self-care decision to make. It helps root you in reality, and takes you out of your I'm-gonna-eat-junk-food trance. It's a wake-up call that kicks you right back on track when you have to answer questions like: *Should I eat that junk food or choose healthy food? Should I keep to my portions or go overboard? Should I get up and take that walk or lounge around on the couch?* In each case, there are only two choices, and each one carries consequences. The target motivation keeps you mindful of the choices and their repercussions so you don't float off and repeat self-destructive behaviors. Bottom line: The target motivation is pretty powerful stuff. Let's help you find yours.

To do that, let's take a closer look at that decision-making process. As in any decision in life, it all boils down to running away from bad decisions that carry hefty prices—financial, physical, and psychological—and steering toward more productive, joyful choices. You have to know what these bad and joyful decisions entail for you when it comes to your self-care. So let's get really personal. First, consider the bad decision.

I want you to conjure up a picture of where you think you'll end up if you don't start taking better care of yourself. Avoid the global motivations. Go deeper. This is a scary place—what I refer to as the "dark place." Many people choose to avoid thinking about this, but it's so necessary to be aware of the driving forces for your behaviors in life. This image will be in your head when you're making self-care decisions and help to remind you to immediately turn away from a bad decision.

I walked Jim, a 48-year-old accountant, through this process. Obese, with high blood pressure, aching joints, and a stressful job, he thought his target motivation was to avoid a heart attack. But that never stopped him from overeating at night. Instead, he went deeper and found his scary vision that of his father: obese, diabetic, unable to care for himself, and dependent upon a walker to get around.

Jim adamantly proclaimed to me, "There's no way I'm going to end up using a walker!" Then we visited a joyful image. He could see himself physically fit, filled with energy, and running after his grandchildren in the park. So here's Jim's target motivation in action: He'd go through his mind-over-mattress dialogue in the morning, and when he chose to get out of bed and hop on the treadmill, he saw himself frolicking in the park. And just in case he had any hesitation, he realized that the walker was waiting for him. He'd connected the dots. And, by the way, by sticking to his target motivation, Jim also solved his global motivations. You see, the target motivation leads to the resolution of the global motivations. He was soon off his high-blood-pressure medications, his knees stopped aching as he removed his excess body fat, and boy, can he keep up with the kids now!

Karen, a 40-year-old schoolteacher and mother of three, complained of feeling tired and upset about being 30 pounds overweight and unable to fit into any of her clothes. She was shocked when her doctor told her that her blood-sugar levels were borderline high. But apparently none of this was motivating her to stop invading the vending machines in the cafeteria or start lacing up her sneakers for a daily walk. When she did the target motivation exercise, she was stunned to realize that her joy and passion in life was to teach, whether it was her students or her children. What message was she sending them when they saw an overweight, unfit, and unhealthy woman standing before them every day, pontificating about how to live well, and yet not practicing what she preached. She quickly connected her target motivation dots: teacher or hypocrite. Her self-care behaviors would reflect whichever choice she made. She thought of those two words every time she made a self-care decision and was amazed by how much easier it was to stay on track. She's now walking the talk for her students, her children, and herself.

If you have trouble immediately identifying your target words, here's another way to get you there. When you choose appropriately, ask yourself, "Who wins?" Go ahead and say your own name. Mary wins or Frank wins. If you do something inappropriate, the winner is not you, that's for sure. It's that scary image you want to run from, just as Jim and Karen ran from the walker and the hypocrite.

The same applies to kids. The trick is to keep it really simple, doable, and accessible. Kids are highly visual and think in the short term. They need to determine what they really want to do. It could be something like getting into the pair of orange pants that excites them but right now is too tight. There's that "clothes-o-meter" I talk about. Or they simply want to fit in with other kids. Girls and teens want to shop at the cool stores. As boys proceed through adolescence, they want to attract girls, and suddenly the appearance issue takes priority. Heavy kids and teens can get teased and ostracized. That's their scary place. Joy comes from happily hanging out with great friends and participating in fun physical challenges.

One of my most successful kids, Hillary, came to me at 13 years of age. She was already 5'11" and over 280 pounds. I was taking care of her mother who had the same problem (there's that genetics thing again), but Hillary came of her own volition. Here's the deal. I asked her, "What would be the burning desire for you?" In Hillary's case, her global motivations were the obvious: fitting into nice clothes, fitting in with friends, and being able to do more at summer camp. But what about that target motivation?

She said, "I'll be darned if I'm going to go to high school or college looking like this. I need to be healthy. I want to look better. I am not going to college obese." Her scary place hung on the word *obese.*

I said, "Honey, that's fantastic." So in her case, who wins when she makes appropriate choices? With fierce determination, Hillary realized that *she* wins. Her target motivation had to do with a "happy Hilly" or an "obese Hilly." And whenever Hillary said the word *obese,* she ran in the opposite direction. That was the image that scared her into making appropriate decisions. And guess what? It scared 100 pounds off her. Hillary is now 25 years old and has sustained her remarkable achievement for over ten years. She starred in the high school senior play, had a blast in college, and has a great job and a packed social life. (Read more about how she did it on pg 217.)

Bounce Back

The other big "Mind" component is the concept of regrouping. People who do the best on this program are what I call master regroupers. They are stress resilient. Like bamboo in a hurricane, they bend but don't break.

If you need good examples of this idea, the greatest teachers you could ask for are centenarians. The wonderful work done at Harvard Medical School New England Centenarian Study has clearly shown that people who live to be over 100 are often stress-shedders no matter what hits them. And by 100, you've had a few things hit you or you've had no life to speak of! The bottom line is that these people are able to take whatever life throws their way, go through all the normal human reactions like anger or grieving, then just regroup and navigate around the stressors. It doesn't mean that they don't hurt. They just get over it. That applies to their bodies as well as their minds. Something's aching or squeaking on them, but they don't turn it into a second career.

Expect life to happen to you, too. You will have to face adversity. I call it the "reverse-expectation rule." I wake up in the morning, and after I've done my "gratitudes," I say, "Bring it on. Go ahead and let's see what this day brings." You never know what's ahead, and the more rich and complex your life, the greater probability that something is going to happen. Your daughter is diagnosed with ADD; your husband comes home depressed because he didn't get his promotion; the dog chews the antique furniture; your kids get Ds and Fs on their report cards; your mother falls down the stairs and breaks her hip. Just don't let any of it permanently derail you. Simply adapt.

Here are some simple rules to teach you how to improve your regrouping skills:

- Avoid unrealistic expectations, and try not to make assumptions. Instead of using the phrases "I expect" and "I assume," simply say "I hope." That leaves you open to adapt to a wider range of life events. "I hope to get that job" leaves you open to the possibility that you won't, and you're geared up to take action either way. This helps you avoid being blindsided and paralyzed, unable to regroup well.

- Don't take things personally. Life happens, and it's usually more about the other guy's issues than yours. There's lots of projection going on here. Protect yourself from becoming ensnarled in other people's issues, and instead, stay true to your core personal and professional mission statements.

- Turn life experiences and stresses into ongoing learning experiences. As Albert Einstein once said, "In the midst of difficulty lies opportunity." Spend time learning that lesson and using it to improve your life.

- Avoid perfectionism. One of my favorite sayings is "Perfectionism is the enemy of 'done.'" Perfectionism leads to paralysis, which leads to procrastination.

- Let it go. Don't get stuck in the rumination rut. Absorb the experience, learn from it, and move along.

- Arm yourself with wit and humor. You can't laugh and be stressed out at the same time. Opt for humor. It softens the blow of so many life stressors and gives you the opportunity to see life more clearly.

Show how flexible you can be. Don't get paralyzed when Plan A doesn't work. Reality check: Raise your hand if you think your self-care Plan A is going to work for the rest of your life. Of course not. Life is dynamic and constantly changing. Master regroupers realize this and learn to bend and flex, adapting and restructuring their lives to navigate life's stresses and keep on goin'.

One of my patients ran into problems with her home treadmill—it was always on the fritz. She said, "I know what to do every time that stupid thing goes on the blink: go for a walk outside." She's got that master regrouper attitude. So you can't get in a full 30 minutes of walking, but you can get in 15. I love it: When her Plan T (treadmill) didn't work, she made a Plan W (walk). You can learn to do this, too.

During the entire National Body Challenge and beyond, you'll be practicing your regrouping skills. You'll be fighting old self-destructive behaviors and trying out new, healthier ways of living. Attack this Challenge with patience and persistence. For instance, right about the fourth week of the Challenge, the honeymoon period is over and suddenly you realize, "Boy, this is work." This is when many people fall off the wagon. Armed with your target motivation as well as your newly honed regrouping skills, you'll be able to keep plugging along, building that powerful foundation for lifelong health and wellness.

As it becomes part of your life, take your family along for the ride. The wonderful thing about this program is that as you learn and have your own epiphanies, you can share them with your whole family, especially your kids. In this way, you're teaching at the same time you're doing. See one, do one, teach one. Everyone wins!

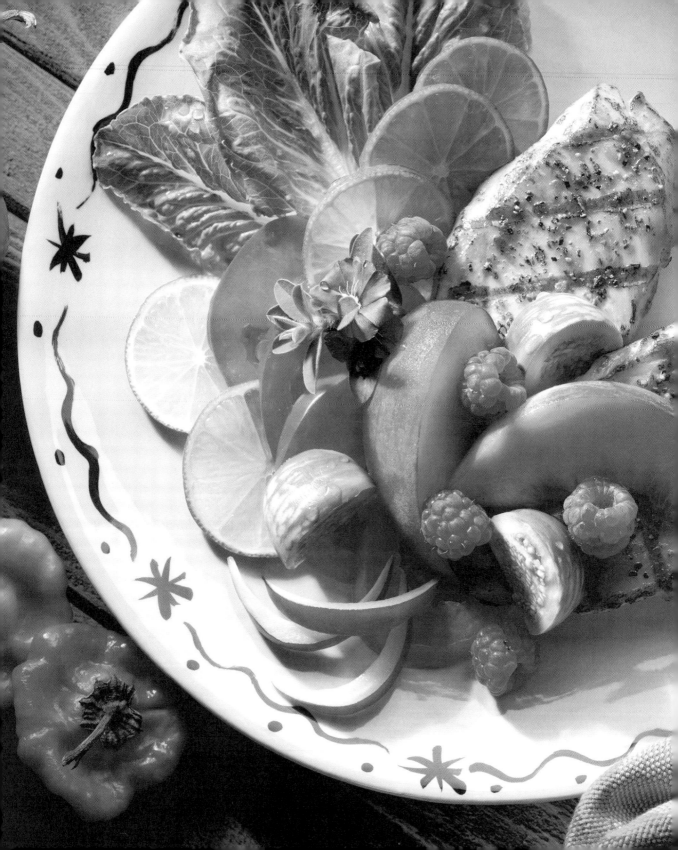

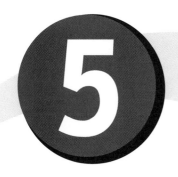

5

Mouth

Thank heavens we're finally entering an era when fad diets are becoming less and less prevalent. Aren't most of you living in a serious state of "been there, done that"? Enough! We're armed with too much great knowledge about nutrition to keep going down that route. There are wonderful scientists working in the field who are teaching us to understand the human body and how simple changes in nutrition work to remove excess fat and keep us healthy.

The National Body Challenge Success Program is all about taking small steps that add up to life-saving changes. And that includes how you eat. Adjust your expectations right now, and don't think that this is about changing your current eating habits overnight. It's one step at a time.

For instance, if you're not a breakfast eater, trust me, you will be before this is over. We'll patiently introduce you to how and why eating a healthy breakfast is one of the chief predictors of success when trying to shed weight and keep it off. We'll also help guide you as you learn how to introduce healthier ways to eat into your daily living. Your goal is to eventually create the healthy eating program that you and your family can sustain for life.

If you're going to be successful on this program, when it comes to food you need to pay attention to three classic elements: quality, quantity, and frequency.

Quality

There are three main food groups or macronutrients: proteins, fats, and carbohydrates. In the past, promoters of fad diets have tried to convince you to eliminate an entire food group. Remember when everyone hopped on the fat- and carb-free diet bandwagons? Science has clearly shown that you don't need to shun an entire food category—just the unhealthy foods within that group. For instance, not all fats are created equal. Olive and canola oils are fats that support a balanced diet; palm and coconut oil, trans fats, and saturated fats do not. So, the key is to go for what I call the "Smart Foods" and grossly minimize or eliminate most of the highly processed and refined foods in each category.

My Smart Foods idea is in line with the newest U.S. Department of Health and Human Services and the Department of Agriculture's Dietary Guidelines for Americans (**www.dietaryguidelines.gov**) Food Pyramid recommendations for both adults and kids. See it at **www.mypryamid.gov**. Experts now agree that we need to minimize or eliminate refined and processed foods in our diet and prioritize whole foods like fruits, vegetables, nuts, legumes, and whole grains. You have to train yourself to look for these foods because the others look so tempting, and then customize the pyramid options to work for you and your whole family.

Here's an exercise for you to do together: Next time you shop for food, take the family to the grocery store for a learning experience. Head first for the produce section. There you'll find whole fruits and vegetables: the Smart Carbs. Then, just for an exercise, avoid going down the aisles and just walk the perimeter of the store. Take a good look around. Usually, you'll see dairy products, whole grains, prepared foods in the deli, as well as frozen foods: plenty of Smart Proteins, Smart Fats, and more Smart Carbs. Now saunter down the aisles and be aware that the processed foods you see requiring bags, boxes, and cartons are not whole foods. Of course there are some healthy foods here (canned vegetables, oatmeal, nuts), but pay attention to those foods chock full of table sugar, processed flour, added fat, and sodium.

These foods have gone through a manufacturing process whereby most if not all of their nutritive value has been depleted, leaving you with a product that not only has empty calories, but may even be harmful to your health as well. Most fat-free desserts are loaded with refined sugar that increases your risk of diabetes. Frozen pizzas are filled with hydrogenated, trans, and saturated fats that can elevate your risk for high blood pressure, heart disease, and stroke. Pizzas, take-out Chinese foods, processed meats, and some canned foods are high in sodium, which can cause you to bloat and, in people who are sodium-sensitive, can increase the risk for high blood pressure. Check your sodium intake with the handy calculator on Discovery Health Channel's Website: **http://discoveryhealth. com/tools/nutrition/sodium/sodium.html.**

Here's a simple rule to help you choose healthier foods. When in doubt, eat my Smart Foods. They're the whole foods that will give you great macronutrients—as well as vitamins, minerals, and antioxidants. Antioxidants neutralize free radicals, which may damage your body's cells and promote ill health and aging. Smart foods also satisfy you more than processed foods and will fuel all the great physical activity you're going to be doing. You can find more choices on the Smart Foods Chart.

Smart Protein

cheese
 cottage, ½ cup
 light or fat-free hard cheese, 2 oz.
 ricotta, ⅓ cup
eggs, 1
egg whites, 3 or 4
egg substitute, ⅓–½ cup
fish, 4 oz.
 catfish
 haddock
 salmon
 tuna
 shellfish (shrimp, crab, lobster)
meat, 3–4 oz.
 skinless chicken
  or turkey white meat
 lean beef or pork
 lean deli meat

soy foods
 "chicken" patty, 1
 "burger," 1
 "hot dog," 1
 "cheese," 2 oz.
 soy milk, 8 oz.
 soy nuts, ¼–½ cup
 tofu, 4 oz.
 yogurt, low-fat, 8 oz., dairy or soy

Smart Carbohydrates

vegetables 1/2 cup cooked;
 1 cup raw
artichoke
asparagus
broccoli
Brussels sprouts
cabbage
carrots
cauliflower

Smart Carbohydrates (cont'd.)

- celery
- corn (starchy)
- cucumber
- green beans
- mushrooms
- onions
- peas (starchy)
- pumpkin
- radicchio
- romaine lettuce
- spinach
- squash
- sweet potatoes (starchy)
- tomatoes
- zucchini

Fruit
(1 whole fruit or 1 cup berries or melon chunks or ½ cup cooked/canned or ¼ cup dried)

- apple
- apricot
- blueberries
- cantaloupe
- grapefruit
- nectarine
- orange
- peach
- pear
- raspberries
- strawberries
- watermelon

Whole Grains

- barley, ½ cup cooked
- brown rice, ½ cup cooked
- oatmeal, ½ cup cooked
- whole-wheat or multigrain bread, 1 slice
- whole-wheat bagel, English muffin, pita bread, or wrap, ½
- whole-wheat pasta, ½-1 cup cooked

Smart Fats

- avocado, ¼
- canola oil, 1 Tbsp.
- nuts
    - almonds, 15
    - peanuts, 20
    - walnuts, 12
- olive oil, 1 Tbsp.
- safflower oil, 1 Tbsp.

Junk Food:
Grossly Reduce or Eliminate

- candy bars
- chips
- cookies
- full-fat red meat
    - steaks
    - bacon
    - ribs
- full-fat cheese, yogurt, and milk
- ice cream
- pastries
- processed meats
- bologna
- hot dogs
- sausage
- white sugar
- white pasta
- white rice
- white bread
- most crackers
- buttery popcorn
- soda

Make up three meals a day by having one serving of protein, one serving of carbohydrates, and half a serving of fats. For two of those meals, make sure to have an extra serving of a nonstarchy vegetable from the Smart Carbohydrate list. In addition, have two snacks a day.

Confused about how to put it all together? See the following for some sample menus for breakfasts, lunches, dinners, and snacks. You can also find loads of great quick and easy recipes using these foods that the whole family will enjoy on the Discovery Health Website at **http://discoveryhealth.foodfit.com**. If you register for the Challenge—which runs between January 14 and March 11, you'll receive access to a week-by-week meal plan that includes over 200 recipes and over 300 meal choices.

SAMPLE MENUS

Breakfasts

- Whole-grain cereal mixed with ½ low-fat milk and ½ plain yogurt, topped with ½ sliced banana, and cinnamon.

- Whole-grain bagel spread with fat-free cream cheese and all-fruit spread.

- 1 light English muffin, toasted and filled with 1 slice light Swiss cheese, a thick slice of tomato, and fresh basil; 6 fl. oz. low-sugar orange juice.

- Hot oat-bran cereal (¼ cup dry cooked with 1 cup skim milk) with raisins, sprinkling of brown sugar or sugar substitute, and cinnamon.

- 100- to 150-calorie drinkable yogurt, 1–2 slices whole-grain toast (plain or with light coating of trans-fat-free spread).

- Store-bought protein shake or make your own (2 scoops protein powder, 1 frozen banana, 1 fresh peach, water, skim milk, or soy milk, unsweetened cocoa powder. Blend on high for 5–10 seconds). Have half now and refrigerate half for tomorrow.

- 1 egg or equivalent pasteurized egg product, 1 tomato sliced, grated fat-free mozzarella cheese over all; 4 oz. blueberry juice.

- High-protein cereal (10 or more grams per serving) with low-fat milk and topped with fresh berries.

- Whole-grain waffle with light syrup, a large spoonful of cottage cheese, and kiwi slices.

- 1 slice French toast made from whole-grain bread, 1 cup diced melon, cherries, and a few pecans.

- Breakfast pilaf (½ cup cooked) and 1 scrambled egg or egg substitute; 4 fl. oz. calcium-fortified orange juice.

- Soy sausage, ¼ cup cooked brown rice, and orange slices; 4 fl. oz. tomato juice.

- 150-calorie bran muffin and 1 hard boiled egg; 10 fl. oz. low-sugar cranberry juice.

- ½ cup fat-free ricotta cheese combined with ½ cup applesauce or crushed pineapple (no sugar added), sprinkling of cinnamon and slivered almonds.

Lunches

- Quick quesadilla (1 low-carb, high-protein tortilla drizzled with olive oil and topped with 1 whole roasted red pepper, grated low-fat mozzarella or feta cheese, and sprinkling of dried mixed herbs). Top brown for 5 minutes.

- 4 oz. salmon with cucumber and dill salad (1 cup thinly sliced cucumber mixed with ¼ cup minced red onion, ¼ cup nonfat plain yogurt, 2 tsp. vinegar, 2 tsp. fresh dill, salt to taste).

- Fresh spinach salad with 3 oz. diced chicken breast, fresh strawberries, poppy seeds, and a splash of orange juice.

- ½ cup brown rice stirred into ½ can store-bought lentil soup, 1 slice crusty whole-grain bread.

- ¾ cup whole-grain pasta (wheat, rice, corn, or quinoa) with stir-fry vegetables (snow peas, broccoli, red pepper, carrots, straw mushrooms).

- 1 fat-free whole-wheat pita and dip (¼ cup hummus and ¼ cup low-fat cottage cheese); fresh fruit of choice.

- Brown rice salad (½ cup cooked brown basmati rice mixed with lightly blanched celery, sugar snap peas, carrots, and scallions seasoned with fresh or dried herb mix). Serve atop fresh greens.

- Mexican wrap (low-carb, high-protein tortilla filled with sauteed green and/ or yellow squash, mushrooms, onions, peppers, and seasoned black beans). Glass of low-fat dairy or soy milk.

- 1 slice whole-grain bread spread with 2 Tbsp. guacamole, a few baby carrots, baked chips.

- Mixed vegetable chowder (corn, tomatoes, beans, and winter squash thickened with mashed potatoes, seasoned to taste and garnished with fresh parsley).

- Minestrone soup with ½ sandwich (1 slice whole-grain bread, fat-free lunch meats such as chicken, turkey, or ham; low fat Swiss cheese, and piled high with lettuce and baby spinach).

- Pita pocket stuffed with roasted portobello mushroom and any of the following: roasted red pepper, spinach, fresh tomato, Vidalia onion, scallions, reduced-fat cheddar cheese, garlic, or cilantro.

- Spicy black bean veggie burger on whole-grain bun with no- or low-calorie ranch dressing and topped with generous portion of sprouts, tomato slice, and fresh basil.

- ½ cup seasoned brown and wild rice mixture atop chopped fresh green pepper, red leaf lettuce, shredded purple cabbage, mixed fresh or dried herbs, splash of fresh lemon juice and olive oil.

Dinners

- Sirloin kebabs and Mediterranean vegetables (small red onions; red, green, orange bell peppers; large mushrooms). Thread 3 oz. meat cubes and vegetable on skewer and brush with marinade. Broil/grill 8–10 minutes.

- Ground turkey stew (brown turkey then mix with garlic, onion, chopped fresh or frozen vegetables, and cumin). Serve with side salad.

- 4 oz. salmon topped with nonfat yogurt and dill; roasted carrots, green salad.

- ½ breast baked chicken Parmesan; green beans; fresh tomato and cucumber salad (1 cup thinly sliced cucumber mixed with 2 tsp. vinegar, 2 tsp olive oil, 2 tsp. fresh dill, salt to taste).

- Vegetarian lasagna (low-carb, high-protein lasagna noodles, low-fat cheeses, precooked eggplant, onions, mushrooms, spaghetti sauce). Large green salad.

- 4 oz. stir-fried shrimp with Asian vegetable medley (snow peas, carrots, broccoli, pearl onions, bok choy; seasoned with a few drops of sesame oil, garlic, and fresh ginger root).

Snacks

- Yogurt with flax meal, wheat germ, dried fruit, or nuts.

- Light string cheese with apple, orange, or kiwi.

- 8–10 almonds with ¼ cup raisins.

- Light popcorn.

- 1 Tbsp. nut butter with celery or apple slices.

- Whole-grain crackers with hummus.

- Whole-wheat English muffin topped with seasoned tomato paste, grated fat-free cheese, and toasted.

- Low-fat deli meat rolled up in lettuce leaf.

- Soy nuts with high fiber cereal and a few raisins.

- 100- to 150-calorie drinkable yogurt.

Start smart by considering the color of your diet. Is it primarily white? If so, it's time to add some color. Hang around in the produce section of your grocery store and look at all the fresh fruits and vegetables in a variety of colors you'll find there. The deeper and richer the color of your produce, the higher levels of nutrients and antioxidants they contain. Forget about that washed-out iceberg lettuce. How about trying radicchio or those marvelous red peppers, deep green spinach and broccoli, orange and yellow squashes and sweet potatoes? If you do, you'll be getting your daily requirements of vitamins A, B, and C, along with life-giving minerals such as potassium, magnesium, zinc, and selenium. Let's not forget tomatoes. They have lycopene, which is a very powerful antioxidant that seems to lower risk for some cancers and heart disease. You men, especially, listen up: Lycopene is extremely important in prostate health; it has been found to actually impact prostate cancer in a positive manner.

Please go for fruit in a major way. Try for balance and variety. I don't mean that you should have five bananas a day. How about an occasional pear or nectarine or some melon? It's all good stuff. I happen to be a berry fanatic; mixed berries really work for me. They also have great antioxidants. Strive for five servings a day, but do remember, though, that all these foods have calories. (You'll learn about servings and portions in the next section.)

I don't care if you choose fresh or frozen produce. Frozen is fine because almost all fruits and vegetables are frozen immediately after they've been picked and retain high levels of their nutrients. When it comes to lycopene, you'll get the best bang for your buck from cooked tomatoes, so add them into wonderful soups and sauces.

The other parts of the grocery store to haunt are those aisles that have grains, cereals, and breads. Color comes into play here, too. Always choose the darker products over white ones. Why? The white breads, unlike dark breads, have been made from processed ingredients so that most of their nutrients are now gone. In the bakery area, go for multigrain breads. I'm a real fan of whole-wheat pita, which you can store in your freezer and warm up in the microwave or toaster when you need it. Go for brown rice and whole-wheat pasta, and experiment with grains you might not have tried before, such as barley and quinoa. Pick cereals with low sugar, high fiber, and a variety of grains. Kashi, Mueslix, and oatmeal are great choices.

All these whole grains as well as fruits, vegetables, and beans are higher in fiber than processed products. And a diet rich in fiber is helpful with weight management. It fills you up with fewer calories and helps you feel satisfied between meals. There are health benefits, too. Science shows that fiber-rich foods can decrease your risk for colorectal cancer and also plays a part in the treatment of diabetes because it slows the absorption of glucose. So are you getting enough? Find out with the tool on Discovery Health Channel's Website at: **http://discoveryhealth.com/tools/nutrition/fiber/fiber.html.**

When it comes to protein, hold back on the fattier red meat cuts, which are heavy on saturated fat. Instead, choose the leanest cuts of beef and pork (look for "90 percent lean" on the label) and skinless white-meat poultry. Put fish on the menu at least a couple of times a week, and choose from wild salmon, tuna, haddock, catfish, or shellfish. Egg whites and pasteurized egg substitutes are great sources of protein, and so are nonfat yogurt, skim milk, cottage cheese, and other low-fat cheeses.

Don't forget your legumes or beans, as they provide protein when combined with whole grains. You vegetarians (and you nonvegetarians who want a change), stock up on soy foods such as tofu, meat and cheese substitutes, soy milk, soy chips, protein powder, and energy bars. Women—especially peri- and postmenopausal women—might try to introduce soy into their diets. It's a great source of protein as well as calcium. Women need 1,200 to 1,500 mg of calcium daily to maintain strong bones, and many don't get enough. Check your intake by using the tool on the Discovery Health Website: **http://discoveryhealth. com/tools/nutrition/calcium/calcium.html.**

Fats are an essential element of our cells. Go for the Smart Fats by replacing mayo and butter with healthy, monounsaturated oils—olive and canola. Nuts like almonds and walnuts and nut butters (peanut or almond) are other good sources and make great snacks. Avocados provide monounsaturated fat in a really tasty form.

Feeding Kids and Teens

I want to put in a special word about kids here. The goal is to provide your children with a balance of Smart Foods along with the occasional treats. It's exceptionally important to remember that they're growing astronomically and they must have appropriate amounts of Smart Foods plus vitamins and minerals to support that growth. Just make sure to get fruits and vegetables in their food along with appropriate protein all day long. As best you can, make certain that sandwich has green things in it; when you're making that soup, put in loads of vegetables. Combine fruits with yogurt to make a parfait: Kids love that; it tastes great. The USDA has found that the majority of children have so little input of vitamins and minerals that sometimes the only ones they get are fortified cereals in the morning—if they even have breakfast at all.

If your doctor looks at your child's growth chart and notes that he or she is overweight, you need to regroup and assess what kinds of foods you're all eating as a family. As a parent, ask yourself what kind of example you're setting by your own eating habits. As you shop and prepare foods for your family, particularly limit the amount of processed foods with high contents of refined sugar. Soda is a huge problem. Studies have shown that 50 percent of teenage boys are drinking at least three or more sugared sodas a day. And each one may have the same amount of caffeine as two to three cups of coffee. Yikes! Try to prioritize fruits and vegetables with high volumes of water and thus fewer calories. This is not so easy to do with finicky appetites and acclimation to high-sugar and high-fat foods. Parents need to be more creative to get kids to enjoy healthy foods. That's where fruit smoothies, carrot juice, and zucchini bread come in.

Change always takes place in small steps. One of the most important things you can do is make sure that your children and teens have a healthy breakfast. Research has shown that kids who start the day off well have a greater chance of shedding extra pounds and keeping them off, as well as doing better in school. Just like adults, kids do well with smaller meals and snacks throughout the day. We'll be addressing that in the Frequency section of this chapter. Suffice it to say, three healthy meals and snacks usually do the trick to keep kids in shape mentally and physically. See page 57 for healthy menu options for kids.

You can help your kids get interested in eating well by introducing them to "My Pyramid for Kids," a section of the USDA and HHS's My Pyramid Website: **www.mypyramid. gov**, which has an interactive game called the Blast Off Game, a tool to make learning about healthy eating and getting 60 minutes of daily activity a fun experience for 6- to 11-year-olds. They'll make choices about what to eat for breakfast, snacks, lunch, and dinner and discover what best "fuels their rocket."

ONE WEEK'S WORTH OF KID'S MENUS

Day 1

Breakfast: Oatmeal, sliced bananas, glass of milk.

Snack: String cheese, apple rings.

Lunch: Sandwich on whole-grain bread with lean turkey and slice fat-free cheese, lettuce, mustard. Baby carrots. Carton of milk.

Snack: Cinnamon graham crackers spread with fat-free cream cheese.

Dinner: Low-carb, high-protein, high-fiber rotini; pasta sauce with meat or of milk. Fresh fruit (grapes, berries, canned pineapple) in gelatin for dessert.

Day 2

Breakfast: Scrambled eggs, whole-grain toast lightly spread with olive oil and Parmesan cheese, 4 fl. oz. calcium-fortified orange juice.

Snack: Low-fat yogurt.

Lunch: Fat-free, 100 percent whole-wheat pita pocket filled with chicken salad made with light mayo, minced celery, green pepper, lettuce. Watermelon chunks. Carton of milk.

Snack: Soy chips. "Soda" made from ½ juice, ½ sparkling water.

Dinner: "Pizzas" made from high-protein soft tortillas layered with fat-free mozzarella cheese, mild salsa, sliced green pepper, canned mushrooms, olives, top browned for five minutes. Mixed salad of greens, tomatoes, shredded carrots, light dressing. One hundred percent frozen fruit bar for dessert.

Day 3

Breakfast: Whole-grain puffed cereal with low-fat dairy or soy milk; 4 fl. oz. grape, cranberry, or blueberry juice.

Snack: Celery stalks and hummus.

Lunch: Macaroni and cheese using whole-grain macaroni and low-fat cheese. Applesauce.

Snack: Granola bar.

Dinner: Three oz. lean hamburger or high-protein veggie burger (optional: on whole-grain bun), roasted potatoes, coleslaw made from grated cabbage, carrots, apples, light mayo or plain yogurt. Three-inch-diameter chocolate chip cookie for dessert.

Day 4

Breakfast: Toasted whole-grain raisin bagel or English muffin with peanut butter. Glass of milk.

Snack:	Trail mix (nuts, dried fruit, high-fiber cereal).
Lunch:	Chicken fajita or wrap, small salad or side vegetables. Glass of milk.
Snack:	A cup of carrots and ¼ cup hummus.
Dinner:	Roasted fin fish or steamed shellfish, mashed acorn squash, seasoned brown rice. Glass of milk. Half cup low-fat ice cream topped with fresh strawberries for dessert.

Day 5

Breakfast:	Whole-wheat waffle spread with light cream cheese and topped with fresh fruit (kiwi, orange slices, mango, etc.), 4 oz. grapefruit juice.
Snack:	Whole-grain pretzels with small box raisins.
Lunch:	Chicken noodle soup, whole-grain crackers, glass of milk.
Snack:	Low-fat cheese-flavored popcorn.
Dinner:	Seasoned black beans and rice, tomato and cucumber salad, glass of milk. A half cup of frozen yogurt with berries and drizzle of chocolate syrup for dessert.

Day 6

Breakfast:	High-protein energy bar (15–20 grams of protein, 4–7 grams of fat, 15–20 grams of carbohydrate) carton of calcium-fortified orange juice.
Snack:	Whole-wheat, banana-nut bread spread with fat-free cream cheese.
Lunch:	Green salad with ½ cantuna, ¼ package of tofu or 2 oz. light feta cheese. Apple, peach, or pear. Glass of milk.
Snack:	Warm cocoa made with milk, sweetened with evaporated cane juice, molasses, or stevia (a natural herbal sweetener).
Dinner:	Baked potato topped with fat-free cheddar cheese, baked beans, steamed broccoli or zucchini, flavored seltzer water. Low-fat brownie for dessert.

Day 7

Breakfast:	Low-fat bran muffin, glass of milk.
Snack:	Cut up raw vegetables (red or green peppers, celery, carrots, sugar snap peas). Low-fat creamy dressing for dipping.
Lunch:	Pasta salad using whole-grain bow-tie pasta, mix of steamed vegetables (mushrooms, olives, broccoli, peppers, carrots, eggplant, scallions), light Italian dressing. Glass of milk.
Snack:	Apple slices spread with 2 Tbsp. peanut butter.
Dinner:	Chili (prepared with ground beef drained of fat, or meatless soy "burger"), beans, chopped green peppers, canned tomatoes, chili seasoning. Half ear corn on the cob with butter substitute. Glass of milk. Ginger snaps or angel-food cake for dessert.

Another great challenge is that kids are eating fewer home-cooked meals today than in previous generations. It's all about take-out and restaurant foods, which are "super-sized" portions, and full of sugar and fats. If you, as a parent, find yourself with no other option than ordering in or eating out, see Surviving the Menu Maze for some helpful tips for navigating restaurants.

And now a word about kids and snacking: The American Academy of Pediatrics has noted that at least 25 percent of children and teens get at least four hours of screen time (which includes TV time, computer time—any type of screen) every day; and that there's a direct correlation between the hours spent in front of a TV and being overweight. Kids are snacking their way through the day, and it's those now familiar culprits: sugary, starchy, refined, and processed foods. It's time to intervene by limiting screen time to no more than one hour per school night and two hours a day on weekends. Then clean up the kitchen and make sure junk food isn't around to tempt them during screen time (or any other time, for that matter).

The 80/20 Rule

Okay, you're motivated and feeling empowered with all of this great information. And so you think your goal is to change everything overnight and to resolve to eat Smart Foods 100 percent of the time. Don't go there. You're doing the "perfectionist thing." This is mostly true of you women. Instead, plan to give yourself a little room for being human, for heaven's sake. You'll be fine if you follow my 80/20 rule. This means that you nail it 80 percent of the time, and give yourself 20 percent flub time. It lends humanity to the entire process.

Surviving the Menu Maze

- Avoid any food option that starts with "fried."

- Stick with grilled, baked, roasted, or charbroiled foods.

- Opt for noncreamy soups that fill you up with all the right stuff.

- Order steamed, roasted, stewed, boiled, or baked veggies.

- Choose the skim or low-fat dairy options.

- Select a regular burger, avoiding the cheese, mayo, and specialty dressings.

- Try chicken or turkey wraps: They're terrific.

- Get your baked potato topped with yogurt, salsa, and/or veggies: It's a winner.

- Avoid white bread: If a sandwich is the only option, just eat the protein that came in it.

- Combine lean protein with salads that have a light dressing.

- When you want dessert, make it fresh fruit, gelatin, or sherbet.

- Hydrate with plenty of water: or how about a flavored iced tea?

- If you have to have a soda, make it decaffeinated and diet.

The Mini Chill

Want to know what a mini chill is? Here's an example. Say you're in an airport, tired, beat up, and enduring yet another plane delay. (I'm in airports all the time—this is something I can relate to!) You decide to have a skim latte in the coffee shop and there's that 140-calorie biscotti sitting right on the counter in front of you. Go ahead, eat it. This is something that you need; it feels good. The Mini Chill only works when you aren't eating what I call a "bingeable." This is any food that you can't have just one serving of without going on a binge. We all know which foods these are. Guys, you know for you it's usually those starches like crackers and chips with dips. And women, for you they can often come in the form of candy or cookies. I'm a jelly-bean-aholic, yet chocolate is no problem. Right now, grab a pen and write down your own bingeables. Then commit to avoiding those foods. They're nothing but trouble. There are plenty of other options.

So, the correct way to do a Mini Chill or treat is to make sure it's not a bingeable. The next rule is to enjoy one serving. Choose it as a true treat. A treat means occasionally. Hey, it's your birthday, so have a piece of cake, for crying out loud. Have some ice cream; just don't have "Mount Saint Ice Cream." There's no reason for you to go overboard. Learn to savor and value your food. That's what a Mini Chill is all about.

And here's another way to make Mini Chills work: Learn to share. You want to have that wonderful dessert on the restaurant menu? Fine. Ask who else wants to share it with you. This will guarantee that you don't eat the whole thing.

Go back to any time you were learning something new. For instance, think back to when you first tried to drive a stick shift. You hit that 100 percent of the time, didn't you? No! You crunched that thing—a lot. Watch your own children as they learn in school. Are they perfect? Of course not. Don't ever lay that kind of a trip on them. At school and on this program, just say, "Hey, honey, do the best you can," and with practice and patience as well as watching you "walk the talk" at home, they'll get it. By the way, don't ever tell a child something's healthy. There's only a minority of children who will get the health connection. Most will run the opposite way. Try to say, "Wow, these taste good" or "This is so much fun to make, come on and help me out," and many of them will accept that. Engage and empower them with participating in the process of choosing and preparing healthy foods.

The Mouth part of the program is like anything you learn in life: There are days you're going to hit it 100 percent, or even 150 percent; then there are the days you'll hit it 50 or 60 percent. But successful people consistently average 80 percent. It's funny how that works. And what comforting news.

Quantity

Now that you know to choose Smart Foods, just how many calories' worth of them should you eat? Well, this is all about avoiding the land mines of portion distortion and sticking to healthy serving sizes. What do I mean by this? Over the past ten years, soda, burger, and fries sizes have become three to five times larger than they used to be. We're living in a "super-size" nightmare. A small cup of soda today was the regular size a decade ago. We have to retrain ourselves to reject these ridiculous oversized food portions and learn what's appropriate for ourselves and our families.

Realistically, you can approach the issue of quantity by choosing Smart Foods, and then either counting calories by simply watching portions or a combination of both. It's perfectly fine if you want to start off by just choosing smarter and eating appropriate portions. Refer to the Smart Foods charts and serving recommendations and stick to those. Eventually, though, everyone needs to learn what a calorie is, and honor the fact that all foods have calories, and eating too many results in weight gain.

You don't have to obsess about calories. But just like shopping for anything, it's smart to know the "price" of each food item you choose so that you can balance it with your "currency" (daily physical activities) and maintain a healthy weight. At some point, everyone needs to learn how to read a food label (see page 64) and determine how "expensive," or calorie-dense, certain foods are, and where the real bargains are. (They are in watery fruits and vegetables, of course!) Most experienced healthy eaters get very savvy about what the "high ticket" items are and either avoid them, or plan to work them off with exercise.

A calorie is a unit of energy. It's the amount of fuel you get from the food you eat. It gives you the energy to walk up those stairs, run after the kids, or hoist your groceries into the car. Everyone needs a baseline amount of calories to maintain their current weight. Once you know how many calories you need, you can either maintain the status quo, increase them to gain weight, or decrease them to shed pounds.

Once you know the approximate number of calories you need, it's like a daily nutritional budget. Like monitoring your checkbook, you have limits and boundaries you need to adhere to if you want to achieve your healthiest body composition. What does your budget look like?

We're going to ask you to estimate the number of calories you need to be eating a day. There's a little bit of math involved here, but you can do it.

> 1. Figure out how many calories you burn when you're simply resting quietly and doing nothing more than breathing. This is called your Resting Metabolic Rate (RMR). To find it, multiply your current weight by one of the numbers below. (See Chapter 2 to estimate how far above the normal range for weight you are.)

> *If you are:* 10–30 pounds overweight multiply by 10
> 31–50 pounds overweight multiply by 9
> 51 pounds and up overweight multiply by 8

> *Your RMR =* _____

2. Figure out how many total calories (TC) a day you need to stay as you are now. Multiply your RMR by one of the numbers below depending on how physically active you are *currently* (not how active you intend to be on the Challenge).

If you are: Sedentary—do no physical activity other than daily chores, multiply by 1.2

Minimally active—do 20–30 minutes of non-intense physical activity three times a week, multiply by 1.3

Moderately active—do 30–45 minutes of moderately intense physical activity five or more times a week, multiply by 1.4

Very active—do one or more hours of intense activity ever day, multiply by 1.7

Your TC = _____

3. Decide how much weight per week you want to remove on the Challenge, and then figure out your daily calorie requirement to achieve that goal. Be realistic, now. From your TC, subtract a calorie amount depending on how much weight you want to remove.

If it's: Half a pound a week, subtract 250 calories
One pound a week, subtract 500 calories
One and a half pounds a week, subtract 750 calories
Two pounds a week, subtract 1,000 calories

Your daily calorie requirement = _____

Please note that you're not supposed to cut all those calories from what you eat. I suggest that you reduce your food intake by half that amount and then burn off the rest with physical activity. So say you want to remove one pound a week, reduce your calorie intake by 250 calories per day, and do 250 calories' worth of additional daily physical activity.

The next thing you need to know is what those calories should consist of. I'd like 20 to 30 percent of them to come from fat. Really, 25 percent is your goal. If you eat too much fat, you wear it. Connect *that* dot! And remember, I'm talking about Smart Fats. Aim for having less than 10 percent of your total fat intake come from saturated fat. You might not realize just how much saturated fat you're getting in animal protein and prepared and packaged foods. There's a useful tool on the Discovery Health Website to help you figure that out: **http://discoveryhealth. com/tools/nutrition/satfat/satfat.html**.

For protein, the range is anywhere from 15 to 25 percent. You cannot build muscle if you're not getting enough protein. Women tend to undereat it. They should be getting about one gram per kilogram of body weight. That's a minimum of about 60 to 80 grams of protein a day for an average-size woman. More physically active and muscular women or athletes have different nutritional requirements and need to take in at least 100 grams of protein. But you really have to go out of your way to do that.

Most men are pretty good at getting in their daily protein. If anything, many of you overeat it big time. Eating half a cow and a pound of bacon are poor quality and quantity decisions. So pay attention to Smart Proteins (poultry, fish, lean red meat, soy, legumes, skim or reduced-fat dairy) and portion sizes. When in doubt, men, eat half of what you normally eat. With experience, knowledge, and refining, you'll get the hang of appropriate eating for guys.

With Smart Carbs the range is 50 to 60 percent of total intake, with the majority coming from vegetables, secondarily from fruit, and third, from the multigrains. Carbohydrates are what will fuel all that magnificent physical activity you're going to be doing every day. When, indeed, you don't have enough energy to get it done, you're probably not getting enough carbohydrates. But as with fat, overeat carbohydrates and those extra calories are converted into fat and you'll wear them.

That's all well and good, but you're probably now wondering what all those percentages and grams actually look like on your dinner plate. The grand majority of you have absolutely no clue about portions and servings of food; but it's not your fault. Growing up you probably ladled food onto your plate. I certainly

Shake It Up

I've got a tip that's good for everybody: males, females, and kids: Make shakes. Get some whey or soy protein powder in vanilla flavor. One scoop of the powder will give you about 20g of protein. Combine it with skim or low-fat milk and fresh or frozen fruit, and you have yourself a phenomenal protein shake.

For you women, shakes are a great mid-afternoon snack when your energy is beginning to drag. Protein is especially satisfying, as it increases the feeling of satiety, so after your shake you'll be good to go for it least three hours. It will definitely cause you to be less hungry at dinner time. So by doing this, you won't overeat in the evening, which is a guarantee for weight gain and also for skipping breakfast in the morning.

did. There were five kids, and I was always battling it out for food with brothers who outweighed me by a whole lot and were much taller than me. Now when you eat out you're usually presented with enough food for a whole family in one serving.

So here's the deal: I didn't know about portions either. I had to start reading USDA food labels and wipe the shock off my face when I found out that a serving of brown rice is half a cup. Look at the table on this page. What you see is an example of a USDA food label that is on every type of packaged food in the grocery store. This is important: I want you to start reading these labels on every food item you buy. Now come on, don't give me that look. When you buy a sweater, don't you read the label to see if it's wool or cashmere and why you're paying all those bucks for it? Well, it's cashmere, for heaven's sake! You certainly wouldn't buy a car without reading the labels. This is a no-brainer, so I'm going to teach you how to read food labels.

The first things you'll see when you look at the label are the serving size and the number of servings in the package. Serving sizes are usually provided in cups or pieces. Like me with the brown rice, you'll be surprised to find out just how small many serving sizes are. Now, next time you're in the grocery store, compare the serving sizes of cereals. You'll notice that very often the serving size of those sugary, high-fat, low-fiber cereals is half a cup. But the serving size of the smart multi-grain, low-sugar, high-fiber cereal is one cup. You get twice the amount of food for a similar calorie count. Interesting, isn't it?

Once you become a regular label reader, you'll also get "sticker shock" from the number of servings. How many times have you bought a bag of potato chips or trail mix and downed the whole thing in one go? Look at the label and you'll discover that you've been eating anywhere from five to eight servings, maybe even more! This applies across the board: A serving size of soup is half the can, not the whole can; a serving size of a frozen pizza is one-third, not the entire pie.

Nutrition Facts

Serving Size 1 cup (52g/1.8 oz.)
Servings Per Container About 8

Amount Per Serving

Calories 140	Calories from Fat 10
	% Daily Value**
Total Fat 1g*	**2%**
Saturated Fat 0g	**0%**
Trans Fat 0g	
Cholesterol 0mg	**0%**
Sodium 85mg	**4%**
Potassium 480mg	**14%**
Total Carbohydrate 30g	**10%**
Dietary Fiber 10g	**40%**
Soluble Fiber 1g	
Insoluble Fiber 9g	
Sugars 6g	
Protein 13g	**20%**
Vitamin A 0% •	Vitamin C 0%
Calcium 6% •	Iron 10%
Phosphorus 20% •	

* Amount in Cereal. One half cup of fat free milk contributes an additional 40 calories, 65mg sodium, 6g total carbohydrates (6g sugars), and 4g protein.
** Percent Daily Values are based on a 2,000 calorie diet. Your daily values may be higher or lower depending on your calorie needs:

	Calories:	2,000	2,500
Total Fat	Less than	65g	80g
Sat. Fat	Less than	20g	25g
Cholesterol	Less than	300mg	300mg
Sodium	Less than	2,400mg	2,400mg
Potassium		3,500mg	3,500mg
Total Carbohydrate		300g	375g
Dietary Fiber		25g	30g
Protein		50g	65g

Calories per gram:
Fat 9 • Carbohydrate 4 • Protein 4

Next, you'll see the number of calories in one serving, and how many of those calories come from fat. Say there are 200 calories in one serving and 50 calories are from fat. At a quick glance, that might not seem unreasonable to you, but if you haven't noticed that there are two servings in the box and eat the whole thing, you're eating twice as much as you think you are: 400 calories, including 100 calories from fat.

Underneath the calorie count is a list of nutrients starting with fat and ending with protein. Here's where you find out how much of your daily allotment of fat, carbohydrates, and protein you're getting from this particular food. Fat is further broken out into saturated fat and, starting in January 2006, trans fats. These are listed separately because science shows that they raise LDL ("bad") cholesterol levels that increase your risk of heart disease. It makes sense, then, that you'll want to avoid products containing high servings of these fats as much as possible. The same goes for the cholesterol. Also, look at fiber and sugar amounts. Given a choice of two similar products, go for the one with higher fiber and lower sugar.

Below the nutrients is a list of micronutrients such as vitamins and minerals. Some fortified products like juice, bread, or cereal will have a long list. You particularly want to make sure you're getting the "big four" vitamins: A, C, D, and E.

If you want to find out a whole lot more about the food label, and even quiz yourself on your knowledge of it, go to **http://vm.cfsan.fda.gov/label.html**. Or, check out Discovery Health Channel's web interactive on the food label at: **http://discoveryhealth.com/centers/nutritionfitness/interactives/foodlabels.html**.

So there you are with your half-cup serving of brown rice. It sure doesn't look like a lot when you put it on a plate, does it? The trick is to add *volume* to it by piling on foods like vegetables that have a lot of water in them. Put a whole stack of vegetables next to your brown rice, sprinkle on some shredded low-fat cheese, and what you've got is visually a lot more satisfying. You've got yourself a happening thing. Trust me. This will fill you up well.

Also, learn the fine art of tasting. Science shows that the best tastes come from the first two fork- or spoonfuls. Eat slower, savor that food, and share it. Suddenly it takes much longer to eat, and you'll find you need less. For an interesting exercise, try a meditation dinner. Set up a beautiful table, complete with favorite foods, in a lovely room, and have soothing music playing in the background. Just concentrate on the food—its appearance, smell, feel, texture, and taste. Don't be surprised if you eat slower and consume fewer calories. You'll be too busy enjoying it to wolf it all down mindlessly while talking to three other people and/or watching TV. It's all about paying attention to the sensual experience eating should and can be. And, it's a great way to keep portions in check.

Bottom line: Be aware of portion size, portion distortion, hidden labels scams, and super-sized offerings. If there's a specific food that you like, simply check it once and learn what a serving size looks like. Soon measuring out that portion will be second nature. To get you started, look at the chart on the next page.

Food Portions

Food	Size of
Rice or pasta	A lightbulb
Baked potato (5 oz.)	A computer mouse
Bagel (½)	A hockey puck
Muffin	A large egg
Meats	Your palm
Nuts	A Ping-Pong ball
Butter	The tip of your thumb
Cheese	Two dice
Raw veggies (1 cup)	Your fist
Cooked veggies (½ cup)	A lightbulb
Fruit	A tennis ball

Frequency

We recommend that you eat roughly every three to four hours starting with breakfast. There's good science showing that people who abide by this principle achieve and maintain lower body fat levels, are able to sustain them with greater ease, and feel satisfied throughout the day. For most people this is going to be breakfast, mid-morning snack, lunch, mid-afternoon snack, and dinner. Sound like a lot? Raise your hand if you've ever had a kid. Was that kid hungry every nine hours? Wrong. He or she was hungry about every three to four hours, and if he didn't get fed you had that "wah-wah" thing going on. That's a primal cry of hunger. Think back to being a child yourself. You knew what hunger felt like. You'd say, "Gosh, Mom, I'm hungry, it's lunchtime." That's what you want to get back to.

Here's a thought: Children are teachers, too. They can take you back to your roots and reteach you what you should have remembered all along. But, oh boy, you got kind of mixed up along the way. We still feel the hunger but as adults we blow it off because we just have too many other things going on.

You may be afraid that eating so frequently will cause you to eat too much because you have a big appetite. There's a difference between hunger and appetite. Hunger answers the question, "What do I need?" The answer to that is, "I need food. I'm shaking, I've got a headache, and I've got funny noises in my tummy." Hunger is a visceral, biologic, physiologic event that speaks to need. Appetite, on the other hand, answers the question, "What do I want?" It's a psychological issue. If you put them both together, you have harmony and balance. Healthy, tasty food at appropriate intervals in the day achieves the goal of balanced eating frequency.

Here's what happens when you wake up in the morning nice and hungry and you go down to the kitchen. You say, "I'm hungry and I *need* breakfast. I *want* oatmeal with cinnamon and raisins and some berries and a little coffee." See how it works? Now that's harmonious. You have a nice balance between hunger and appetite. When appetite goes off on its own, you have a problem. Then you have want with no need behind it. That's when you have to have a conversation with yourself.

Want is fine if you're just going to do a mini chill (see page 60). I didn't really need that biscotti at the airport, but I really wanted it. So I had it, and guess what? Nobody died. It was fine, because here's the deal: I exercise, and I stay in fairly good balance, and I'm going to end up making up for that biscotti over time anyway. So every now and then it's fine to give in to appetite. The problem is that most people think they're hungry all the time when they're really experiencing out-of-control, stress-induced appetite, or just have a desire for tempting food. Then, when you eat all day, you never give your body enough time to feel hungry, so you lose track of that primal hunger feeling. It becomes a vicious cycle.

What does this actually look like in terms of how you eat? See page 51, and you'll find menu ideas laid out very clearly so you can see how women, men, and children eat. Here's an important point: You can't eat on a regular basis unless you plan to do so. What I teach my patients is: "If you fail to plan, you plan to fail." So ritualize the day you go shopping for food, take the foods you need to work for your snacks and meals, and try not to leave yourself empty-handed when hunger hits. You need to do this for your kids' lunch and meals, and you need to do this for yourself as well. It's part of ensuring you achieve your healthy daily lifestyle goal.

Also refer to the sample food log we gave you in Chapter 2, and right from day one, start filling in your own logs. But why do you need to do this? This is an easy way to stay accountable. Also, you're a scientist at the University of You. If your name is Jane or Jim, you're taking Jane or Jim 101. Everyone has patterns, and you're learning all about yours. Men often leave hours between lunch and dinner, come home and voraciously eat a bacchanalian feast. Women are more apt to have tried to eat a mid-afternoon snack, but often choose incorrectly (bag of pretzels, vending machine fare), and by the time they get home from work, they're off and running. They overeat dinner and keep things going even while in bed. Then you have the typical American *menage a trois*: you, Ben, and Jerry. Who was the crazy person who said there were four servings in a pint of this stuff? Ask any hormonally challenged woman with PMS or in perimenopause, propped up in bed watching television, tablespoon in hand, if this makes sense!

Some women start overeating at 3:00 P.M. because they may be in contact with the kitchen and kids coming home from school. It's also a time when you have a decrease in your energy and you find you're overwhelmed, exhausted, and lacking focus. If you're at work and one more phone call comes through, you're going to hurt somebody. The next thing you know the vending machine is calling to you. This is when you go back to your target motivation and use that "appropriate and inappropriate" technique. But if you're eating with frequency and keep an appropriately sized whole-food snack on hand, you'll make it through what is perhaps the toughest part of the day. And you'll make it through this program, too.

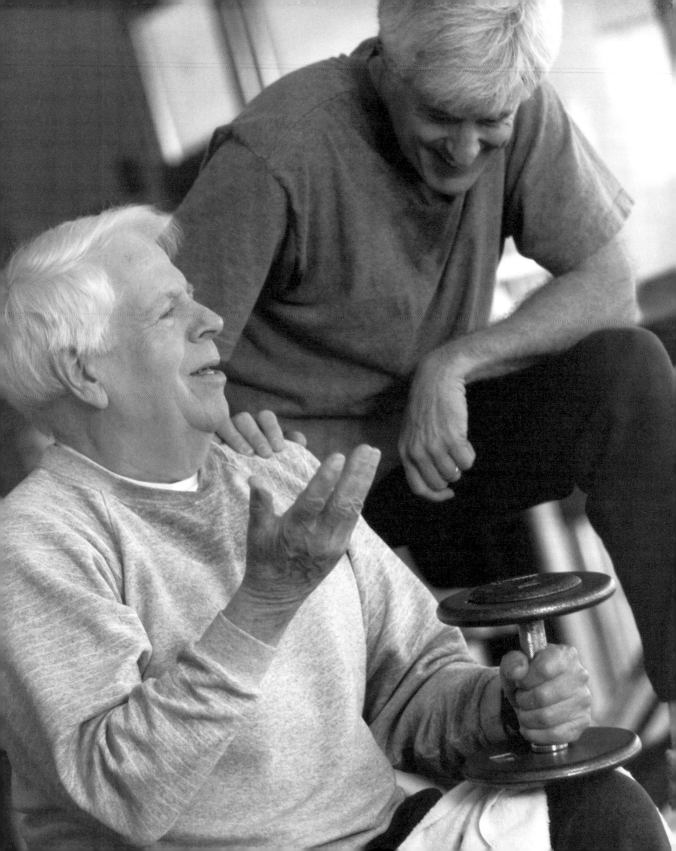

6

Muscle

By now you know that in order to get healthy, you need to do your mental homework and get focused. That's the Mind component. And, you've read how to integrate Smart Foods and healthy eating into your lifestyle. That's the Mouth part. The third and final step is to keep the focus going and burn the calories you've been eating throughout the day. That's the Muscle element.

It's all about keeping a simple balance: What goes in (food) must come out (physical activity). If it doesn't, you wear those extra calories! In science, we call it the Energy Balance Equation. This Muscle chapter shows you the role your physical activity plays in keeping you in balance as you get and stay healthy.

The first rule is that in order to *remove* weight, we have to *move* weight. But unfortunately, we're living in a society that's all but eliminated the opportunities to move. Dependence on automobiles, remote controls, computers, cell phones, elevators, and lack of parks and walker-friendly sidewalks are just some of the elements contributing to our sedentary lifestyle.

Worried parents keep their kids at home, afraid of kidnappings or dangerous neighborhoods. Health clubs are often pricey, and most don't allow minors to participate. We used to turn to schools for salvation here, but no longer. In 1995, physical activity in schools accounted for 18 percent of a child's exercise. Today, it's less than 10 percent, as schools have all but eliminated this class as a required part of the curriculum. And remember those wonderful after-school teams and sports? Now, due to financial crunches, many schools charge parents for their kids' participation, leaving many cash-poor families with no recourse.

Finally, as adults have adapted to higher lifestyle expectations, two working parents has become the standard, leaving little time for their own physical activity, let alone creating family time to get up and move. However, fear not. We're going to show you that despite these challenges, you can still get active.

Moving your body is a natural, normal phenomenon and must be integrated into every single day of your life in one way or another. In our sedentary world, we have to create the opportunities; we can't wait for them to happen unless we have a very physically active job. It's important to understand that the cutting-edge science here is not the E word, "exercise"; it's all about the P and A words: "physical activity." We're looking for what the National Institutes of Aging calls "activities of daily living." It's no longer mandatory to hang out in a gym to achieve your activity goals (although you can certainly supplement your daily physical activities with gym workouts if you want to and have access). You can get in loads of activity at home, work, and in between. Gardening, biking with the kids, and carrying your own groceries to the car are all simple ways to do it. Every little bit counts. A walk here, taking the stairs there, and by the end of the day you've met your activity goal. So the great news is that anyone, anywhere, can make this work.

In fact, we just need to fidget more. An interesting 2005 study of physical activity using movement detectors showed that slender and fit people averaged up to 350 calories more of fidgeting and physical movement throughout the day as compared to those who were overweight. Think that's not much? Well, not doing that can result in your gaining about 40 pounds per year. Now are you impressed? So join the lean and the restless and you'll be burning more calories.

Create opportunities to move. Since society isn't providing you with these opportunities, you have to be resourceful and find them for yourself. This is especially true for families. Doing the National Body Challenge is a perfect chance to share this experience with the kids. On weekends, take the family on a picnic and throw a ball or a Frisbee. Ride bikes or go swimming together. Go for a walk with the baby stroller. Find out what the kids like to do and sign them up for classes. Ask them if it's ballet or martial arts that will kick-start their enthusiasm. Heck, just stick to home base and play jump rope, shoot hoops in the driveway, or how about playing hide-and-seek or tag? When it comes to kids, it's so important to infuse lots of fun into the activity so that they look forward to doing it again and again.

Here's another rule: Physical activity has to be a *nonnegotiable* part of your family's life. Remember that word. It means that there's no option. It's not for just when you feel like it or you're in the mood for a wellness binge. Moving is essential to healthy living, and it's got to be incorporated into your daily living.

Keep in mind that the goal is to minimize body fat, while you strengthen and tone your muscles. If you recall, your metabolism is influenced by genetics, thyroid function, and muscles. By now you're aware of the power of genetics, and you know how to monitor your thyroid function. But the biggest opportunity you have to influence your metabolism is by keeping your muscles in great shape. They'll be the calorie-burning engine you need to remove the fat and boost your metabolism.

The formula for success involves a combination of cardio and strength training. The good news is that there are many options to choose from. Just as you did in your Mind and Mouth templates, you'll be using these options to customize your physical activity as well. This has to work for you and your family. Get ready to experiment. Through trial and error, you'll discover what's doable and realistic. Let's get up and start to move more—right now!

Can-Do Cardio

Cardio activities are all about burning up your fuels—both sugar and fat—as you engage in a variety of physical activities that help keep your heart in great shape. Hence the word *cardio,* short for "cardiovascular" or "heart-centered." Walking, running, skipping, hopping, stair climbing, biking, rowing, swimming, tennis, and hiking are all examples of activities that need oxygen from the air you breathe in order for you to perform them well. That's why another word for these cardiovascular activities is *aerobics.* Cardiologist Dr. Kenneth Cooper coined this term over 30 years ago while he was developing the first programs encouraging Americans to get up and move more to improve heart health.

To see how many times your heart has beat and how many breaths you've taken over your lifetime, click on Beats and Breaths at: **http://health.discovery.com/tools/calculators/beatsbreaths/beatsbreaths.html**. You'll gain a new appreciation for how hard your body works for you and why you should make every effort to keep it healthy. Kids will get a kick out of seeing this, too: They'll be blown away by the numbers.

As well as being important for maintaining cardiovascular functioning, cardio activity, of course, also helps remove the excessive fat that increases your risk for heart disease, cancer, and diabetes.

What's our recommendation for you? If you're a beginner, you need to phase in physical activity over time, and allow your body to adapt to increased daily movement. Start out by buying a pedometer to measure how many steps you take. Simply clip it on your waistband and go about your normal daily activities. Before going to bed, look at the total number of steps you took. The average for most Americans is about 4,000 steps. Your goal is to walk 10,000 steps or more per day. There are about 2,500 steps per mile, so you'd be walking about four miles throughout the day. You burn roughly 100 calories per mile (for a 150-pound person), so 10,000 steps will result in a daily calorie burn of about 400.

Research has shown that 10,000 steps is an effective, proven way to remove excess fat and to sustain your weight removal. For that matter, results from the Weight Control Registry Study from the University of Colorado have shown that of the 4,000 adult participants who've removed 50 pounds or more and kept it off for ten years or more, most accrue 400 calories of activity every day to sustain their weight removal.

Whatever your starting point, just add 500 to 1,000 steps per day, and practice this for a week; then ramp it up another 500 to 1,000 steps per day until you reach your 10,000-step goal. Don't obsess about hitting 10,000 every single day. You may accrue 15,000 to 20,000 on busy weekend days, and 6,000 to 8,000 on more limited weekdays, so it will average out over the week. Your heart loves it when you take it out for exercise. And every step you take goes toward preventing medical conditions and, if you already have them, toward getting off high blood pressure or diabetic medicines.

If you've already been doing some cardio, shake up your routine. How many years has it been since you hopped on a bike or strapped on roller skates? Have you explored all the cardio equipment at your gym, such as the elliptical trainer, stair stepper, or rowing machine? How about trying a Spinning class? What you liked last year may bore you this year, so experiment and be adventuresome and find something new to fire up your enthusiasm.

How often should you do your cardio? The new Food Pyramid Guidelines recommend that you try to get in at least 60 minutes of some form of cardio exercise every single day. I understand that juggling time is a struggle for many people and families, so I'm recommending that you try to do cardio at least five days a week. This goes for kids as well. When you do, ramp up the intensity if possible so that you keep trained and on target. It's something I call Vitamin I = Intensity. As you get in better shape, you can burn calories more efficiently and engage in more challenging aerobic activities.

What that entails is working in the upper end of your target heart rate zone. Target heart rates are based on your age and represent a range, such as 114 to 152 heartbeats a minute. The lower number is 60 percent of the fastest heart rate that a healthy person of a particular age should have during exercise; the high end of the range is 80 percent of the fastest heart rate. Once you've been exercising for a while, you may be able to aim for this higher end of the range, and that's where intensity comes in. The fastest heart rate, also called maximum heart rate, is the highest safe heart rate for your age. You'll find a tool for calculating your own target heart rate zone at **http://discoveryhealth.com/tools/calculators/hrc/hrc.html**.

If you happen to be of an age where you have some disability issues—your weight-bearing joints hurt—then navigate around that problem. Remember about regrouping and stress-shedding? So what you want to do is find some way to get in your cardio activity. Try swimming or water aerobics, and learn to jog or briskly walk in the pool. Experiment with the recumbent bikes at your gym. All of these things help tremendously. See what works for you, and customize your program. For a variety of cardio activities along with the calories you'll burn, go to the Activity Burn Rate Calculator on the Discovery Health Website. Click on **http://discoveryhealth.com/tools/calculators/activity/activity.html**.

What's the goal for kids who need to shed some pounds and get fit? They need to accrue at least one hour of higher intensity activity per day. This is a recommended part of the Department of Agriculture Food Pyramid, and kids will learn about it when they go to the **MyPyramid** site (**www.mypyramid.gov**). Since most schools have little or no physical education programs, you have to be assertive about making sure your kids are getting it.

One key ingredient to success in getting kids up and moving is making it fun. Mix it up and challenge them to do lots of activities. Another key is ritualizing physical activity for them. Games and sports are part of this. Investigate your local community for classes, programs, and clubs where your kids can participate with other children in everything from swimming to martial arts and sport leagues. But just getting up and playing around randomly is a terrific way to get kids addicted to how good physical activity can feel. Encourage your children to get out and play more *and do it with them.* That's right. If they see you just sitting around, they'll do that, too. I know I sound like a broken record, but you are their mentor, and they need your guidance. If they learn this now, they will keep it going as teens and adults.

Teens are a challenge. High schools have almost no PE classes anymore, so today's teenagers are less likely than previous generations to get any activity on school days. While boys are often concerned with their appearance and are more likely to spend time in a gym, physical activity falls off dramatically for teenage girls. Other than athletic girls, most stop moving much, just as body image and sexuality issues come to play. This is the most important time for girls to stay active. Again, find something that your teen might want to do. Tennis lessons, skiing, hiking, dancing, and walking clubs are good starting points. The truth is that if your teenager is currently overweight and nobody intervenes to help, there's an 80 percent chance that he or she will become an obese adult. That's sobering news and a call to arms to every parent out there. Show them you care by guiding them through your own example and support of their efforts to become more active.

Hey, and remember that when you move your body, you're moving your mind as well. Physical activity is such a wonderful way to experience the mind-body connection. And talk about a win/win! Science has clearly shown that when people of all ages, kids as well as the aged, just get up and move more regularly, they think more clearly, their mood is elevated, they handle stress better, and their memory is sharper. Kids do better in school as exercise beneficially impacts upon the learning process. Feeling down? Take a walk—a walking meditation—and you'll see that at the end of it, you may not have solved the world's problems, but you'll feel that you can better cope with them.

Strength Training for Life

Why do you need to weight-train at all if you're doing all that cardio? While cardio is helping burn excessive fat and build aerobic performance, resistance training helps maintain the integrity of your muscles, which represent your main lean tissue mass. This is important, because as muscle becomes more trained, it becomes more effective at burning calories. So, cardio or aerobics burns fat, and strength training builds a stronger, more powerful engine to burn even more fat calories.

Picture a car. You start the engine and begin driving. You're burning the fuel in your gas tank to move the car. That's the cardio. How *fast* you burn that fuel depends upon how powerful your engine is. If you have a racing car with a large engine, you're burning up that gas a heck of a lot faster than if you had a little economy car with a four-cylinder engine. So, I'm telling you to aim for being an 18-wheeler here, not some little ol' car choking up the hill. It's power we need and power you'll get from strength training! How much do you need? Classically, twice a week does the trick quite nicely. That means you're doing your cardio every day you can, and on the days you do strength training you're also getting in your cardio.

Check out the exercise program that follows this page. What you'll see are simple ways to be able to do your strength training even if you have some disability or decreased functioning. In fact, these exercises concentrate on increasing your ability to function no matter what your age. You want sturdy arms to haul those groceries, or a strong back and legs to be able to bend over and lift your grandchild. If you're a new parent, you'll need to be physically powerful if you're going to be throwing a baby stroller into that van on a routine basis. You cannot caregive someone else if you cannot get out of the chair yourself.

Getting out of a chair essentially is a "squat," and you need strong quadriceps muscles as well as hamstrings and calves to do it. If you're in your 50s or even over 60, this is a perfect time to build strength to maintain your independence. This is very important, especially for women, who like to preserve their strength and care-giving skills throughout their entire lives.

Just as with cardio, you can also customize your strength-training program. Try some new things and work them into your routine to shake it up. Have you ever tried yoga or Pilates? Both increase your strength, mobility, and flexibility. How about core work (it strengthens your back and abdominal muscles): We show you some of these exercises on page 79. Maybe take a class or two at the gym.

Flexibility

As you get older, in additional to cardiovascular health and strength, flexibility and balance become very important. Around the age of 40, our ligaments that attach muscle to bone become drier, and that's what contributes to our inflexibility. Therefore, it's important to keep ourselves "well greased," as it were, in order to maintain our flexibility. In addition to which, after the age of 40, something's going to hurt! That's just a fact of life. This is especially true if you've been athletic earlier in your life and you feel those creaks of osteoarthritis coming on. Even if you haven't been athletic, this could be nothing more than the cost of weight-bearing over many years. Interestingly, the more physically active you become now, the less problem you're going to have with osteoarthritis. As you begin to move more and more, the pain will become less and less.

Paying attention to balance becomes important after the age of 50. Watch children as they play, teetering on a piece of wood or the curb. See how well they walk across? As you get older, your ability to do that may become somewhat impaired. It's important to stay on top of it. For these reasons, stretching is extremely valuable.

If you're wondering how to fit all this exercise into your life, in Chapter 2 we gave you filled-in exercise logs to give you an example of how it can work. You'll also find the blank daily workout log that you'll copy and fill in every day. As you start the program, you're going to have to make a plan to ensure you get it done. Will you work out at the gym or at home? Are you going to get up early and walk before the day gets out of hand, or do you prefer to do it in the evening to work off the day's stresses? Are you someone who enjoys exercising alone, or do you need a posse to motivate you? Don't leave it to chance. Remember: If you fail to plan, plan to fail.

The Workout Program

As well as ramping up your daily activities in general, you need a specific workout plan if you're going to remove weight and optimize your health. An effective plan involves both cardio and strength training. For the duration of the National Body Challenge program, you'll be doing at least five cardio workouts and two to three strength-training sessions per week. Sound like a lot? You want results, don't you? Be sure to schedule your workouts into your week like any other appointment, rather than hoping to fit them in when you can. Pretty soon it will become an integrated part of your life.

Cardio

A cardio workout is any activity that raises your heart rate for 30 minutes at a time. Adults want to do this at least five times a week. Activities can include brisk or hill walking, running, cycling, aerobic dancing, water aerobics, kick boxing, or using any of the cardio machines in the gym such as the elliptical trainer, rowing machine, or stair stepper. Do something that you enjoy, because that's the activity you'll stick with. Or, if you tend to get bored by routine, mix it up. Doing different activities can also cut down the chance you might get hurt from doing the same repetitive motion.

Be sure to warm up before each cardio session by doing your chosen activity at slow speed or low intensity for ten minutes. This will warm up your muscles and reduce your risk for injury, and also build your heart rate up slowly. Then crank it up for 30 minutes to the highest intensity that's comfortable for you. There's a steep learning curve with cardio: If you keep at it regularly, you'll be surprised by how quickly your conditioning improves. After your workout, cool down by doing the activity at a low intensity again for five minutes to bring your heart rate back down. Then do some gentle stretching. Hold each stretch, without bouncing, for about 30 seconds. If you take, say, kick boxing or spinning at the gym, then warm-ups, cool-downs, and stretching will be part of the class.

Strength Training

Strength-train at least two, and up to three, times a week. Give yourself one day off between strength workouts, so a good schedule would be Monday, Wednesday, and Friday, for example. Each session will last about 30 minutes.

Alternate training the major muscles of your upper and lower body. So if you work out three times a week, train your upper body on Monday, lower body on Wednesday, and upper body on Friday. The next week, start with lower body on Monday, and so forth. Work on your abs after your lower-body workouts. Don't neglect these ab exercises; as well as helping to flatten your belly, they also strengthen your core. A strong core helps to prevent injury and provides a solid, stable base for your entire body.

On the days you train, perform two exercises for each major muscle group. On upper-body days, include exercises that work your chest, shoulders, back, triceps, and biceps. On lower-body days, work your quadriceps, hamstrings, calves, and abs.

When strength training, warm up by doing some light cardio activity like walking on the treadmill for ten minutes before you start working with weights to literally warm up your muscles to lower the risk of injuring them. After your workout, stretch your whole body, but especially the muscles you've just worked.

What You'll Need

You can do this workout at a gym if you have access to one. Should you decide to do the program at home, there's some basic equipment you'll have to get.

Your Home Environment. For those of you who just want to use what you have around the house, you can use canned goods of one to three pounds and substitute these for dumbbells. Fill up pails with water, weigh them, and use them to do your shoulder lifts. I learned that from a patient of mine who owned a dairy farm and had strong and defined shoulder and chest muscles. Lifting logs or compost in the backyard works as well.

Here's another idea: Just use the picnic bench that's sitting out on the patio, or any piece of furniture that will allow you to move about freely and yet be stable. Any solid, stable chair works great to do triceps dips, for instance. Use chairs to balance yourself as you perform simple leg lifts as well as knee bends. A soft rug is a good substitute for an exercise mat. And use your environment well! I like to use any wall to be able to do simple squats by placing my back against the wall and squatting down to a sitting position and holding that for as long as I can. Table legs are great to whip a resistance band around and get a good seated stretch. Learn to be creative, and you can get strong at home.

Dumbbells. You'll need a starting weight that challenges you. You want to be able to do all your reps, but you should be rather fatigued by the time you get to the last couple. For women, this might be 8 or 10 pounds; for men, 15 pounds (but start with the weight that's right for you). If everyone in the family is going on the program, you'll need to get some different-size weights. This is good for you women because you'll have heavier weights on hand when you're ready to increase your intensity. All of you should have three weight sizes so you can do the strength-training exercises by increasing your weight with each set of repetitions.

Prices of dumbbells vary by size and according to what they're made from: There are chrome, rubber-coated, and neoprene dumbbells available. You can get a pair of 10-pound neoprene dumbbells for around $25. Shop around at your local sporting goods store or online for deals.

Incline Bench. Choose one that can be flat or put on an incline. The simplest ones start at around $50. There are some packages available where you can get a bench and a set of weights in varying sizes. Most will cost about $100. This might be ideal if several family members are taking the Challenge.

Resistance Bands. This is great "no-excuses" workout gear. Basically, it's tubing with hand grips, and you can carry it around with you and use it at work or in a hotel room as well as at home. They come in different resistance strengths. They're color coded in yellow, green red, blue, and purple in ascending levels of intensity, so beginners would use yellow, buff athletes purple.

Exercise Mat. You need this for doing floor exercises like crunches and for stretching. It should be spongy for comfort and made from material that you can wipe down when you sweat on it—because you will! You'll find one for about $20. If you decide to try yoga or Pilates, go for a "sticky" mat that your hands and feet don't slide on. They are similarly priced.

The Exercises

Do three sets of each exercise. With each set, increase the weight and decrease your repetitions. Do 12 to 20 reps your first set, 12 to 15 reps the second set, and 8 to 10 reps the last set. For each muscle group, rest for one minute between each set, and two minutes before starting the next muscle group.

Upper Body

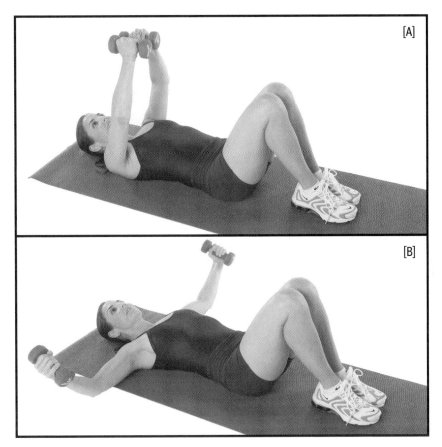

Dumbbell Fly

[A] Lie on the floor, on a yoga mat, with a dumbbell in each hand. Lie back, holding the dumbbells close to your chest. Bend your knees, making sure your feet, hips, and shoulders are pressed firmly against the floor. Press the weights up over your chest with your palms facing together. Keep your elbows bent slightly as though you were hugging a big ball.

[B] Inhale, and keeping the same bend in your elbows, slowly lower the dumbbells out to the sides until your upper arms are parallel to the floor and you feel a stretch in your chest (pecs). Hold for a count of one, then exhale and return to position [A].

Tip: Maintain the same "ball-hugging" shape with your arms throughout the entire exercise. Increasing the bend or straightening your arms decreases the effectiveness of the exercise and puts you at risk for straining muscles.

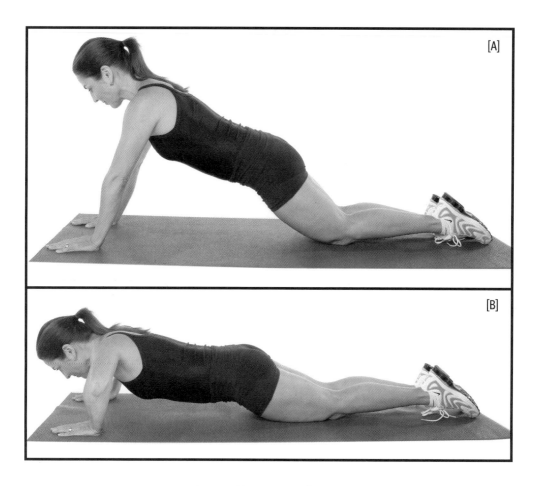

Bent-Knee Push-Up

[A] Kneel on all fours on your exercise mat. Your arms should be straight but not locked and shoulder-width apart, fingers facing forward; your knees should be under your hips. Now, walk your hands forward about six inches, then press your hips forward until your body forms a straight line through your head, shoulders, hips, and knees.

[B] Inhale, and contract your abdominal muscles and squeeze your shoulder blades together and down. Inhale, and maintaining your straight line, bend your elbows out to the sides and lower your torso until your elbows are bent at a 90-degree angle and are aligned with your shoulders. Exhale and contract your chest and triceps, and push up to straighten your arms and return to position [A].

Tip: Don't sway your back. Keep it in a straight line like a plank.

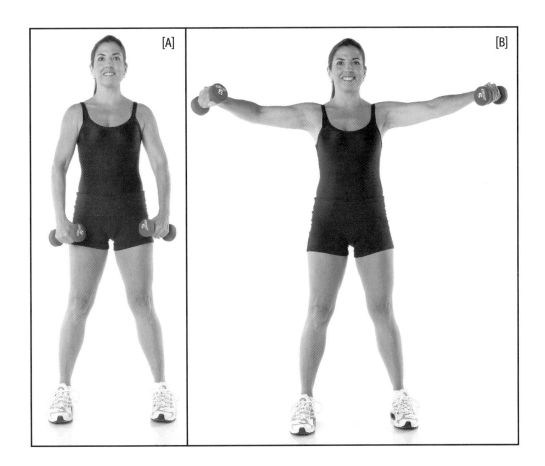

Standing Dumbbell Lateral Raise

[A] Stand with your feet shoulder-width apart, your weight distributed evenly between your heels and toes. Your knees are slightly bent, back straight, and abdominals contracted. Hold a dumbbell in each hand with your arms hanging down at your sides. Your palms should face inward, with thumbs facing forward.

[B] Inhale, exhale, and maintaining your posture, lift your arms up and out to the sides until they're shoulder height and parallel to the floor. Your palms should be facing down. Pause; then inhale and slowly lower your arms to position [A].

Tip: Don't scrunch your shoulders up to your ears. Keep your shoulders down and your chest lifted; look straight ahead with your chin level.

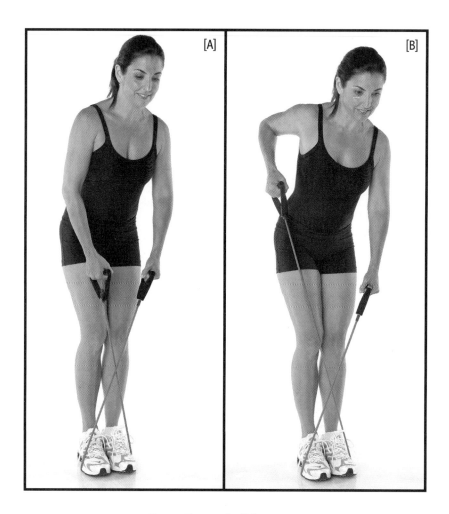

One-Arm Cable Row

[A] Stand with your feet together and knees slightly bent. Place resistance tubing under your feet. Cross the tubing and grasp the handles with your palms facing inward. Bend slightly forward from the waist, keeping your back straight. Press your chest forward and pull your shoulders back.

[B] Inhale, exhale, and retract your shoulder blade to pull your right elbow back and up toward the ceiling. Hold for a count of one, inhale, and return to position [A]. Keep your arm close to your body throughout the movement. After you complete all your reps on the right, switch and repeat on the left side.

Tip: Don't raise the tubing above your mid-abdomen. As you draw back the tubing, it should just brush your side.

Lower Body

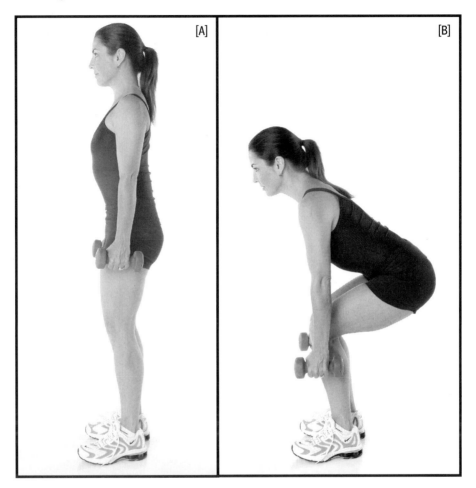

Dumbbell Squat

[A] Stand with your feet shoulder-width apart, your weight distributed evenly between your heels and toes. Your knees are slightly bent, and your abdominals contracted. Hold a dumbbell in each hand with your arms hanging down at your sides. Your palms should face inward, with thumbs facing forward.

[B] Inhale, exhale; and while keeping your shoulders, back, and head upright, bend your knees and lower your hips until your thighs are parallel with the floor. It's as though you were about to sit in a chair. Hold for a count of one, then inhale and return to position [A]. (If you have trouble balancing, try placing a one-inch-thick block under your heels.)

Tip: Keep your back as straight as possible through the exercise, and don't let your knees extend.

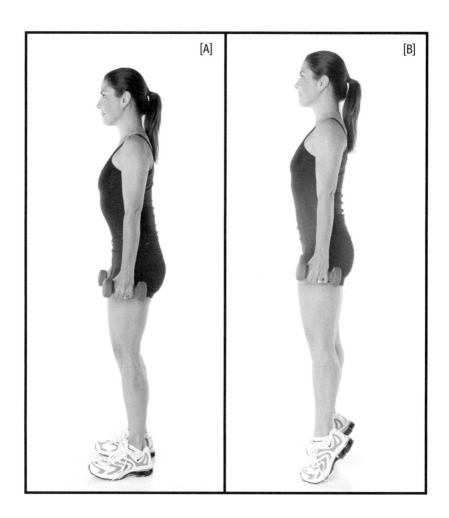

Calf Raise

[A] Hold a dumbbell in each hand, palms facing in, and stand with feet about shoulder-width apart, toes out in a 45-degree angle.

[B] Keeping your legs straight, raise yourself on your toes as high as possible, Pause for a count of one; then slowly lower yourself to position [A].

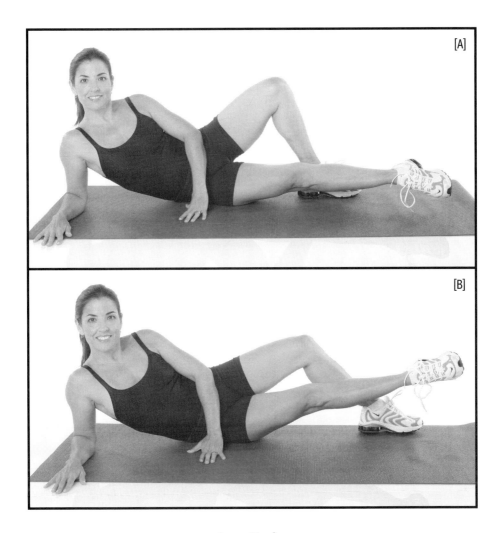

Leg Raise

[A] Lie on your right side and support your upper body by placing your right forearm and left palm on the mat. Extend your right leg straight out a couple of inches off the mat and flex your foot. Bend your left leg and place your left foot flat on the mat behind your right knee.

[B] Inhale, then exhale and lift your right leg up by squeezing your inner thigh muscles. Hold for a count of one, then exhale and return to position [A]. Do all reps and sets on your right side, then turn over and repeat on the left.

Tip: Keep your upper body still; don't use it as a counterbalance to lift your leg. All the work should come from your inner thigh muscles.

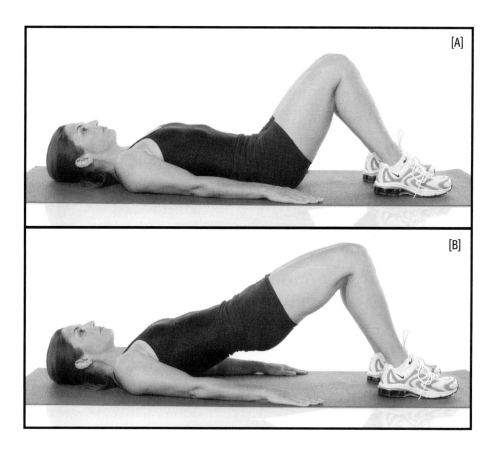

Pelvic Tilt

[A] Lie on your back, knees bent, and feet flat on the floor hip-width apart and about a foot distant from your buttocks. Make sure your weight is evenly distributed between your heels and toes. Place your arms straight down by your sides. Relax your head and neck.

[B] Inhale, then exhale, and push your lower back into the floor and tilt your pelvis up. Contract your abdominal and buttocks muscles and raise your hips off the floor. Squeeze your buttocks for a count of one, then inhale and slowly return to position [A].

Tip: Keep your knees the same distance apart throughout the exercise: don't let them flop in or outward.

Abs

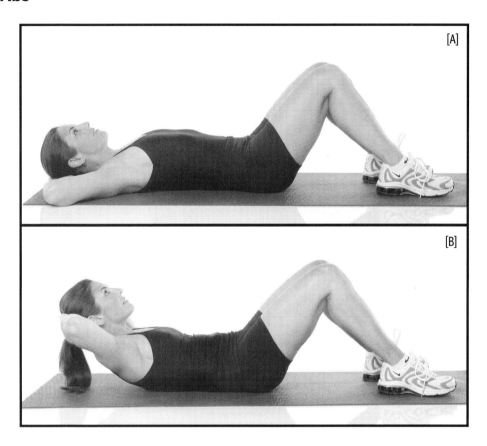

Classic Crunch

[A] Lie on your back, knees bent, and feet flat on the floor about a foot distant from your buttocks. Place your fingertips unclasped behind head, elbows open.

[B] Inhale, then exhale, pushing your back down hard to the floor and rolling your shoulders up, keeping your knees and hips still. When your shoulders are a few inches off the ground, flex your abdominal muscles for a count of one. Then, inhaling, slowly lower back to position [A] without ever letting your back arch.

Tip: Don't lock your hands behind your head or use them to jerk your head up.

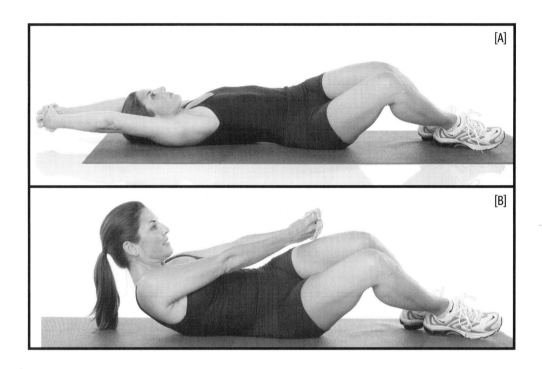

Twist Crunch

[A] Lie on your back, knees bent, and feet flat on the floor about a foot distant from your buttocks. Place your fingertips unclasped behind head, elbows open. Let your legs fall as far as they can to your right side so you're "twisted" with your upper body flat on the floor and your lower body on its side.

[B] Inhale, then exhale, pushing your back down hard to the floor and rolling your shoulders up until they clear the floor, keeping your knees and hips still. Concentrate on contracting the muscles at the side of your waist (your obliques) so that your ribs squeeze toward your hip bone. Hold the crunch for a count of one, then inhale and slowly return to position [A]. After you complete all your reps on the right, switch and repeat on the left side.

Tip: Don't worry if your knees don't drop to the floor. Everyone has different degrees of flexibility.

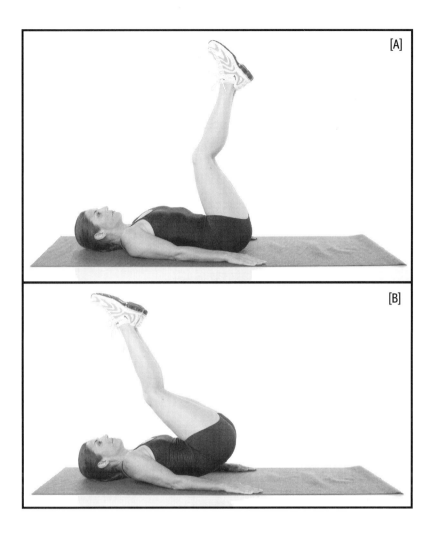

Hip Thrust

[A] Lie flat on your back with your legs straight up at a 90-degree angle to the floor and your feet flexed. Keep your legs straight, but don't lock your knees. Reach your arms behind you and grasp the leg of a bench, table, or any other stable object. Relax your shoulders to the floor.

[B] Inhale, then exhale, and raise your hips up off the floor several inches using the muscles in your lower abdomen to lift them. Squeeze those muscles and hold, then inhale and return to position [A].

Tip: Don't swing your legs over your body. Keep your legs over your hips and your feet directed to the ceiling throughout the exercise.

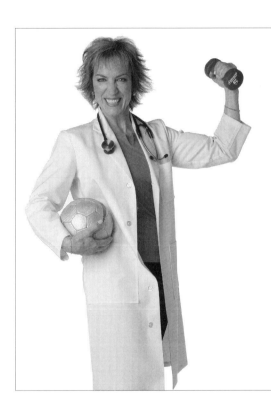

PART
II

**The National
Body Challenge,
Week by Week**

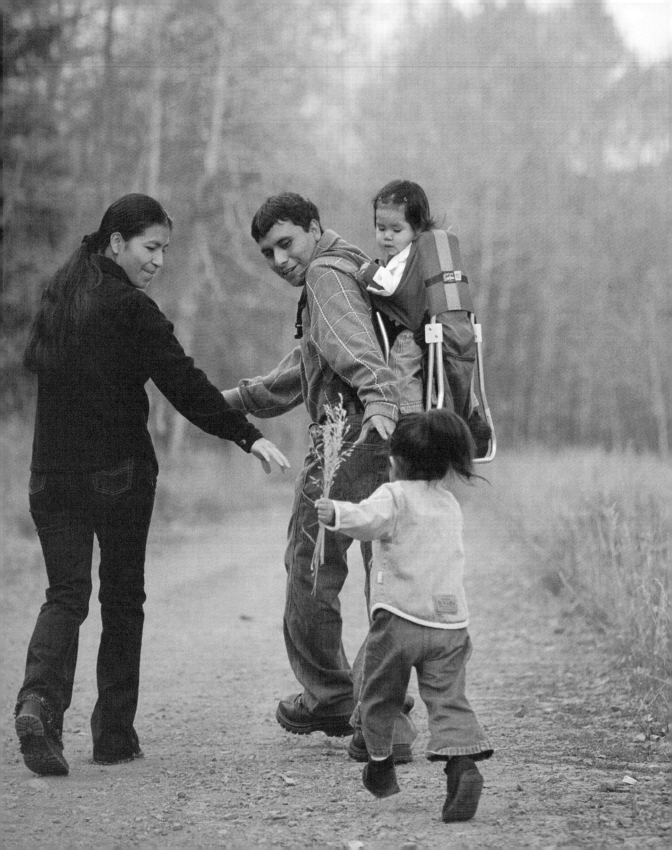

Week-by-Week Rules and Tools for the
National Body Challenge

This Challenge is based upon either an 8- or 12-week Challenge. It's up to you. You can achieve amazing changes in 8 weeks if you put your nose to the grindstone and stay focused. If you want to continue the Challenge for another 4 weeks, feel free. Repeat the whole 8 weeks if you need to.

Whichever way, once you've seen what's possible, the key is to keep practicing your new-found lifestyle habits every day of your life. The National Body Challenge is here to teach you the fundamentals of good nutrition, active living, and stress management. You're using these weeks to learn and hone your skills, share them with your family, and together keep it going.

I'll get you started and then guide you along each week with rules and tools to keep you focused as we troubleshoot potential problems along the way. I developed these over the first two seasons of the National Body Challenge television series based on our work with the shows' participants as well as my weekly chats with all of you across America. We've got tips for the whole family, customized to fit the unique needs of men, women, and children.

Whip out your signed National Body Challenge contract and read it again. Remember your commitment to yourself and your family. As Karen Staitman, a success story from the 2004 National Body Challenge, said after her awards ceremony, "This is the first 12 weeks of the rest of my life." Armed with your own Target Motivation, and filled with the energy to turn your life around, take a deep breath and take your first step. Welcome to the National Body Challenge!

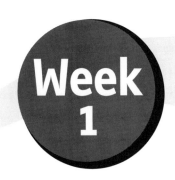

Week 1

Getting *Started*

Walls are built one brick at a time; the same applies to your health. I bet you'll be amazed by how the small changes you start making this week can add up to a major difference in the way you feel and look.

Now remember. If you happen to be a parent, when you get to the kids' part each week, remember to read through this carefully and then get your children to listen to you as you all get active and healthier together.

Little shifts in behavior will accumulate and change your life forever—for the better. So let's go for it!

In preparation, let's make sure that *everyone* has thoroughly read through Chapter 2: Measure Up. Have you done everything you need to do to get off to a running start? Here's your checklist:

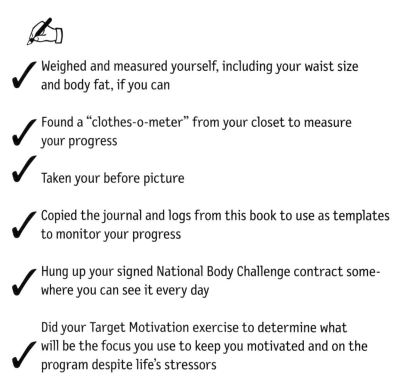

✔ Weighed and measured yourself, including your waist size and body fat, if you can

✔ Found a "clothes-o-meter" from your closet to measure your progress

✔ Taken your before picture

✔ Copied the journal and logs from this book to use as templates to monitor your progress

✔ Hung up your signed National Body Challenge contract somewhere you can see it every day

✔ Did your Target Motivation exercise to determine what will be the focus you use to keep you motivated and on the program despite life's stressors

Now pay attention to the Mind, Mouth, and Muscle elements throughout your Challenge. In your journal, write down your goals in each category. First, you can start with a weight goal. For women, plan on a range of a half pound to two pounds of fat removed per week. For men, it's likely to be from one to four pounds, depending on how overweight you are.

Next, look in each category of the Mind, Mouth, Muscle template and write down up to five goals. Look at the example to see what one 2005 National Body Challenge participant wrote.

Mind

I will:

- Manage my anger better, so that I don't reach for food when I'm out of control.

- Learn how to meditate, and try to practice for at least 10 to 20 minutes each day.

- De-clutter my desk and environment so that I can be better prepared to take care of myself.

- Practice my Target Motivation every time I'm under stress and feel like going back to self-destructive habits.

- Stop taking things so personally and develop a better sense of myself.

Mouth

I will:

- Eat a healthy breakfast.

- Ritualize my grocery shopping instead of winging it every week.

- Plan meals ahead of time.

- Bring my lunch and snacks with me to work.

- Eat every four hours and increase my intake of protein when I do.

Muscle

I will:

- Put my gym bag next to the door to take to work.

- Sign up for spinning classes during the Discovery Health National Body Challenge.

- Buy a yoga tape and try some of the poses.

- Schedule strength training twice a week.

- Try to get my cardio in every day, or at least five times a week.

What you put on your own list are written commitments to yourself. Place them in your journal, and as you accomplish each one, check them off. What a great sense of accomplishment!

Week 1 Rules and Tools

Mind

- Even if you haven't done the preparation above, do as much as you can and take action anyway. Without pondering, ruminating, and "what if-ing," take those first steps that will build your motivation to keep going. Don't put off starting your weight removal and fitness plan a moment longer.

- Make a plan of action for the week. Remember, if you fail to plan, you plan to fail.

- Watch out for perfectionism. Get real. You'll have good days and tough ones. Remember the 80/20 rule.

- Set up your support system—it makes all the difference when the going gets tough. Enlist the entire family, co-workers, and friends who share your interest in maintaining a healthy lifestyle. Together, you can make a run for healthier living.

Mouth

- Choose one thing about your eating to change this week. Eating a healthy breakfast each morning is a great start. Or it could be as simple as preparing some cook-ahead healthy family dinners so you don't have to rely on fast food.

- Be patient. Plan to change your unhealthy habits gradually. Rather then trying to eliminate late-night or after-school junk food binges completely, wean yourself off them by substituting low-fat desserts and snacks and reducing servings to one to two at a time. It won't be easy at first, as your old habits call to you, but stay persistent. It gets easier with each day you practice your new lifestyle.

- Try not to leave more than three to four hours between eating. If you go too long between meals, you'll overdo it when you finally eat. For instance, have a healthy mid-afternoon snack to prevent you from eating too much at dinner.

Muscle

- Simply move more every day. Try my five-minutes-up-per-hour rule. Be fidgety. Find reasons to be active, whether it's volunteering to help others or creating opportunities to move throughout the day.

- Clip on your pedometer. Depending on your current level of activity, aim to add 500 to 1,000 steps every day (for faster results) or every week (for more gradual results) until you reach 10,000 steps a day.

- Check out a health club or community activity center near you for fun classes and challenges.

- Find out about strength-training programs and the availability of trainers to help you learn how to use weight machines, free weights, resistance tubing, and stability balls.

It's a Generational Thing

Kids 7–12

Mind

- Hey, what do you want to do by the end of this Challenge: run, jump, and skip higher . . . fit in with your more active friends? How about getting into those cool jeans you love? Every time it's tough to put down that candy and grab an apple instead, read your journal and remember why you're doing it.

Mouth

- Get on the computer and go to **www.mypyramid.gov** and play the cool Blast Off game. It will help you learn how to pick healthy foods for breakfast, snacks, lunch, and dinner.

- When you wake up in the morning, you haven't eaten for a really long time and your "tank" is empty. You need to fill it up so you don't run out of energy at school. Always eat breakfast. Ask Mom for cereal and milk, whole-wheat toast with peanut butter, or whole-grain waffles and fruit.

Muscle
- Are there kids at your school who jump rope or run around playing games at recess? Ask if you can join in, instead of sitting and watching.

Teens 13–19

Mind
- Get your Target Motivation in focus. Want to go through high school looking and feeling your best? How about really enjoying your college years? Keep those dreams in your mind. Let them guide you to make the right healthy self-care decisions.

- This is a challenging time. Your body is changing, and suddenly it's all about body image and how you're seen by your peers. Just know that living a healthy lifestyle can get you through.

- You're developing from a child into an adult, and the good habits you develop now will last you your whole life. It's easier to start out right than try to correct unhealthy behaviors later.

Mouth
- It's time to pay attention to the sugar issue. Look at how many sugary drinks and snacks you're downing every day. How about substituting water for a soda, or having a low-sugar juice with your lunch or snack?

Muscle
- Even though physical-education classes may be limited in your school, make the most of each class when you're there. Why not sign up for an after-school team just for fun? You need to stay active, as it's all too easy for you to gain weight in your teen years.

20s

Mind

- Adjust your expectations about health and wellness. Don't assume that you still have plenty of time to get in good shape. The key is to lay down a foundation for healthy living *now,* which you can refine during the coming years and which will sustain you for a lifetime.

- Learn how to balance college, grad school, and relationships along with taking care of yourself. Keep your Target Motivation in mind to steer you clear of mindlessness in your self-care rituals.

Mouth

- On-the-go 20-somethings tend to skip meals, especially breakfast. Establish new habits and swear off meal-skipping for the Challenge.

- Become a master of dashboard dining (*but please do not drive and eat at the same time!*). That means learning how to be creative with healthy mobile eating. Make up some trail mix or be certain you have a balanced energy bar available when you're running around with no whole foods close at hand.

Muscle

- Think you'll be bored with just walking? At this age you're full of vim, vigor, and vitality. Change it up by taking a class. How about kick boxing, spinning, or hip-hop dance? There are so many ways to move your body.

30s

Mind

- You're probably busy with career and family. Learn to prioritize and make time for yourself. The best caregivers take care of themselves first.

- Is your Target Motivation to have a healthy pregnancy? Kimberly Dontje (read her story on page 205) did, and she's now the proud mother of a gorgeous baby girl.

Mouth

- You may be preparing food for your family now. This is a great opportunity to assess the quality and quantity of healthy foods in your diet. Start replacing processed foods with whole foods: a piece of fruit for a store-bought muffin, for example.

- As you race around establishing your career, don't forget to fuel yourself with healthy foods every four hours through dinner. Kick the habit of late-night dinners: You'll end up wearing those calories.

Muscle

- To stay healthy and help with stress, make sure to get in at least five cardio workouts a week. Try to do them first thing in the morning before your day gets out of hand. The more complicated your life, the simpler your exercise has to be. Keep track of steps on your pedometer, and record them in your journal.

40s

Mind

- Your body has plenty of surprises waiting for you. Your Target Motivation could be to prevent medical conditions or to reverse one you already have. It's time to take your self-care seriously.

- This is the age when your tummy starts expanding and you need to commit to exercising some "girth control." That extra fat building up inside your abdomen is trouble. It will increase your risk for heart disease, diabetes, and cancer. Watch your waist measurements, and monitor them every four weeks. Women need to get theirs under 35" and men under 40".

Mouth

- You may have spent many years achieving professional success. Now it's time to pay attention to how you feed your body. Find a healthy cookbook, or look for recipes on the Discovery Health Channel's Website, and begin to experiment and customize a food plan that works for you.

- Make an appointment with a nutritionist, and discuss food options based upon your individual needs and tastes.

- Women, supplement with 1,200 to 1,500 mg of calcium fortified with vitamin D for bone health, along with a multivitamin.

- Try to eliminate bread for dinner, and eat starches (pasta, rice, potatoes) in appropriate serving sizes (1/2 cup cooked) no more than three times a week for dinner.

Muscle

- Let your doctor know that you're starting a fitness program. Have a medical evaluation and get clearance if you have orthopedic issues, heart problems, diabetes, or any other condition for which you should be monitored.

- If you haven't exercised on a regular basis for more than a year, be patient and take it slowly as you start your physical activity program. It's easy to be gung-ho and end up hurting yourself.

- If you've been active but doing cardio less than five or six times a week, ramp it up and make your goal five times per week minimum. Cross train and mix it up to keep it fun and lively.

50s

Mind

- Your perspective on health and wellness is changing. Now it's all about disease prevention and treatment. Make your Target Motivation about just being here to enjoy the life you've worked so hard to build. Begin to understand what it's like to live mindfully.

- To age well and maintain your independence, you need strength, endurance, and flexibility. Get a checkup and make sure you know what your limitations may be as you make changes in your physical activity levels and alter your eating.

Mouth

- Fruits and veggies are your natural medicine cabinet. Concentrate on the color of your diet. Eat nine servings a day in a variety of colors. The deeper the color, the richer the store of antioxidants they contain. The aging process is all about oxidation, or how fast the body uses up its cells to keep it going. Antioxidants are great to help neutralize this process and augment a healthy aging process.

- Along with your multivitamin, make sure to take 1,000 mg a day of fish-oil supplements to prevent heart disease.

Muscle

- Physical activity is nonnegotiable. Without it you'll age more rapidly both mentally and physically. Ritualize cardio into your daily schedule. Don't neglect strength training. Men and women lose strength rapidly after 50. You want to build a powerful base of strength and endurance right now.

- Be adventuresome. Try new ways to move your body, understanding that by this age something's bound to hurt and/or not work so well. Give yoga, Pilates, or tai chi a try. Swimming is wonderful for men and women who have arthritis and joint problems.

60s and Beyond

Mind

- This is the time when everyone has one or more conditions that remind them of the need for excellent self-care. You might feels twinges in your back and weight-bearing joints. Your Target Motivation should be to achieve and sustain a strong mind and body, and plan to continue for at least the next 20 to 40 years. It's estimated that by the year 2050, there will be more than one million centenarians. Now that's a great Target Motivation!

Mouth

- You might notice that your appetite and tastes have changed. Reassess the whole foods you eat, and maybe shake it up a bit with newer tastes and combinations.

Muscle

- In addition to your cardio and strength training, pay attention to balance exercises. In your 60s, balance begins to fall off. By combining balance techniques with your routine exercises, you can delay the onset of more serious balance issues.

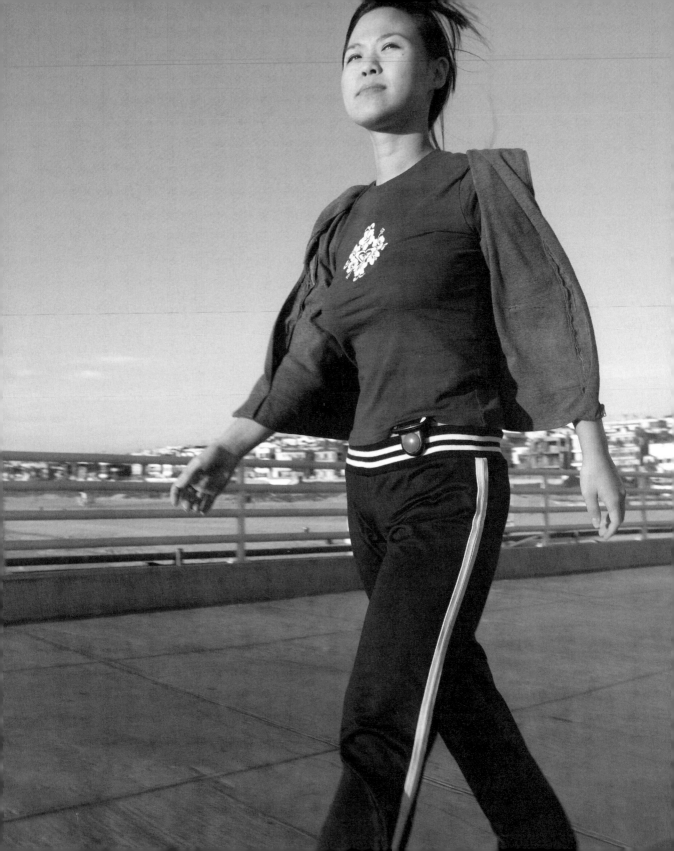

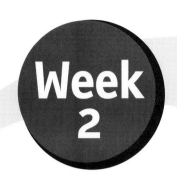

Week 2

Taking It Slow *and* Steady

You've just completed your first week. Quite a learning process, wasn't it? If you've been keeping your journals, you may have had an eye-opening experience discovering that your portions are much bigger than you thought, or that late-night eating is a bear to eliminate. No worries. This is like attending the University of You. You're studying your habits and learning new lifestyle patterns. So let's keep at it.

Week 2 Rules and Tools

Mind

• Don't despair if you made some mistakes in the first week. Look at it this way: In the midst of difficulty lies the opportunity to gain knowledge. That way you have no time for frustration, only proactive learning and progress.

• Don't become overwhelmed by all of the changes you want to make. Last week you chose one thing to modify; do the same now. Perhaps you'll simply take the stairs instead of the elevator. Remember, it's the small steps you make that build the foundation for a lifetime of health and wellness.

Mouth

• Start now getting at least four to five daily servings of fruits and vegetables, and two to three servings of whole grains. Start with oatmeal and fruit for breakfast and you've already got one of each down. Substitute these foods for the junk "white" carbs: table sugar, rice, pasta, bread.

• Add protein to every snack and meal this week: It's the nutrient that fills you up and leaves you satisfied. Protein helps curb carb cravings. Women especially need it. White-meat poultry, lean red meat, fish, and skim dairy products are great ways to get your quota.

• Don't forget the right fat. Olive and canola oils are the best choices. Nut oils are healthy, too. Make a palm-full—no more than 12—of nuts one of your snack choices. Eliminate or minimize saturated fats found in fatty meats and whole dairy products, and some oils like palm and coconut (which, by the way, are used on theater popcorn).

Muscle

• Take your patience pill! Slow and steady wins the race. Continue to phase in your fitness program—especially your weight workouts— slowly to help avoid injury.

• If you've been sedentary for quite some time, you'll notice new feelings as muscles awaken and become trained. That's to be expected. Don't jump in with high intensity. Gradually phase in your weight training and cardio, which will allow your body to adapt. For most of you, this will take from four to six weeks.

It's a Generational Thing

Kids 7–12

Mind

- How does it feel to work together with your family to make your dream of being a happier and healthier kid come true? Remember that it's like being on a team that wants to win.

Mouth

- Help your parents with the grocery shopping. Your body is growing and changing, and this is a really good time to learn about feeding it right so you'll grow up strong, healthy, and able to do whatever you want in life. Learn how to read food labels. Show Mom or Dad how smart you are as you select healthy breakfast cereals, breads, and snacks when you shop with them.

Muscle

- Ask Mom or Dad to let you play outdoors for one hour every day you can. Do it all or once, or you can split it up. Get in one half hour when you come home from school and then another before dinner. Throw the ball with family or friends, get out on your bike, shoot hoops, or just walk and run. Every little bit counts.

Teens 13–19

Mind

- You've got one booked-up schedule as a student and adolescent. Between school and social life, commit to concentrating on one thing you know you can do well—like getting your homework done on time so you're not stress overeating late into the night as you pore over books.

Mouth

- Instead of reaching for fatty chips, cookies, and soda this week, try some healthier snack options such as whole-wheat crackers with low-fat cheese or peanut butter, raisins or dried cranberries, and bottled water.

Muscle

- Scope out some classes you can take at school that will allow you to do some kind of sport or physical activity. Martial arts, tennis, swimming, spinning, dancing, running, soccer, and softball are options. Do something that's fun for you. The key is to keep movin'!

20s

Mind

- Aim to hit your eating and workout goals 80 percent of the time. No one is perfect, and things can happen to make it more difficult to achieve your goals. Do your best given the realistic limitations and constraints of your life.

Mouth

- Watch your portions, even of healthy foods. Remember that a serving doesn't mean a mountain.

Muscle

- How about thinking outside the box? Cross-train with different kinds of cardio activities and equipment. Challenge yourself.

30s

Mind

- When you're juggling work and family, you run the risk of using fatigue as an excuse not to exercise. Try to get to bed no later than 11 P.M. to feel fresh when you wake up and ready for your morning walk or workout.

Mouth

- It's all too easy for distracted parents to pick at their kids' food, or sample dishes while they cook. Watch out for all those extra nibbles; they add up.

Muscle

- Does getting to the gym look like mission impossible with your schedule? Buy some baseline equipment—dumbbells, exercise bands, a yoga mat—for your home. Get some workout videos, maybe weight training, Pilates, yoga, or some form of cardio movement such as Tae Bo. It's like bringing the gym to your home, and the entire family can use them.

40s

Mind

- Are you discovering that it's not as easy to get into the swing of things as it was when you were 20 or 30? The 40s usher in major changes in body composition and metabolism. Self-care is nonnegotiable. So nix the excuses, get serious, and get this journey going.

Mouth

- Your metabolism won't let you overeat and get away with it. Late-night snacking is especially problematic. After 5 P.M., eliminate or minimize your starch intake (bread, pasta, rice, potatoes). Concentrate on salads, veggies, protein, and fruit.

- Introduce soy-based products into your diet. They're a good alternative to animal protein, as they contain no saturated fats are lower in calories, contain dietary fiber, and can help lower cholesterol.

Muscle

- Ramp up the intensity of your workouts. Get some hills into your walking. Lift slightly heavier weights. Do yoga for better flexibility as you age.

Mind

- Persistence and consistency in your attitude and lifestyle habits are essential elements of success. Don't let unrealistic expectations creep into your head. This is no overnight miracle. You're aiming for a sustainable and meaningful mental and physical transformation. And you're gonna do it!

Mouth

- Energy bars and drinks are great for men and women who want a snack or meal replacement in a pinch. Look at the label for this macronutrient balance: 150 250 calories, 4–7 grams of fat (1–4 grams of saturated fat); 10–25 grams of carbohydrates; 10–25 grams of protein.

Muscle

- Buy the right shoes for walking to keep your feet in great shape. Get fitted for shoes by experts at a sporting-goods store. Women, you can buy men's shoes, too. They often have better padding and come in wider widths.

- Invest in some sessions with a personal trainer. It will help you get on an appropriate and customized workout routine. Get recommendations from friends or from your health club for someone who specializes in working with mature clients.

60s and Beyond

Mind

- You probably have more time than before to devote to taking care of yourself. You have windows of opportunity to walk, visit the gym or community center, and engage in group sports (golf, hiking, biking, swimming). Make the most of these precious times to increase your wellness and decrease disease health risks.

Mouth

• Now that you have the time to socialize, be cautious about the extra calories you're ingesting during the cocktail hour and at dinner. Routinely have just one glass of wine no more than two or three times a week. Make hard liquor an occasional drink, as it has far more calories than wine and tends to leave people open to overeating.

Muscle

• You've got more time to travel. Plan an active vacation that allows you to use your mind and body to their fullest potential. Schedule this for six months or more from now. Then, keep training to meet your goal to hike, bike, kayak, or mountain-climb somewhere wonderful and perhaps exotic. You deserve the joy and thrill of this achievement.

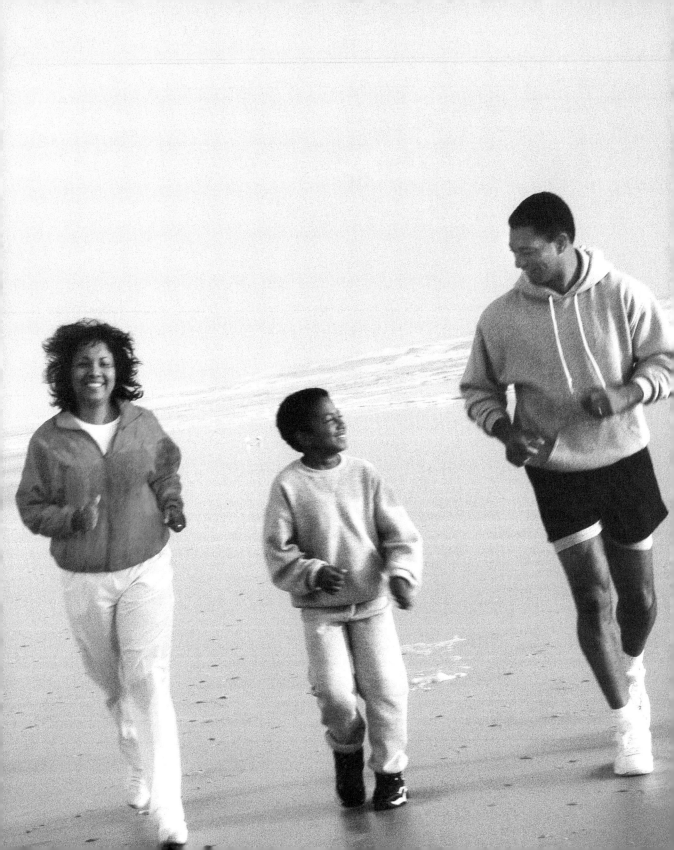

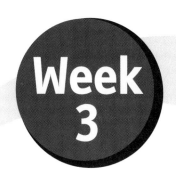

Combating
Stress

Have you noticed a pattern as you've progressed through Weeks 1 and 2? Just when you think you have this new lifestyle under control, something happens and you find yourself saying, "You know, I was doing just fine until [fill in the blank] happened." It could be anything from a brutal deadline at work, to a relationship crisis, to the diagnosis of a medical condition.

But, you know, life is filled with these kinds of challenges. The toughest obstacles in life are the daily stress-inducing events that can distract you from your health goals. You need to expect them and be ready to regroup. That's the essence of good stress management.

Realize that staying physically fit helps you stay mentally fit and more capable of handling life's challenges. This is a win/win proposition. You can do this!

Week 3 Rules and Tools

Mind

- When stress blindsides you the next time, stop and take five deep abdominal breaths. Make each inhalation and exhalation last as long as you can. Breathe in through your mouth and out through your nose. You can do this anytime, anywhere.

- Use your head. That's right—try meditating. It's great for stress management. Listen to tapes, CDs, or take a class. Or just start by sitting comfortably and closing your eyes in a quiet environment for just a few minutes. Work your way up to five to ten minutes at a time. Many people start out the day with meditation, but it's something you can do at any time.

- Pick up the phone and vent to a friend. Better yet, find someone to take a walk with you. There's nothing like a walk and talk to reduce stress, help you think more clearly, and control stress-induced overeating impulses.

- Create calm environments at home or work. Keep some soft music on in the background, paint your walls in soothing colors, use muted lighting, and try some calming aromatherapy scents like lavender for a spalike experience.

- Organize your life—say, your desk or kitchen. Nothing causes stress like poor time management and a cluttered, muddled life. Break a large project into small, doable tasks. You'll feel better immediately. Start now—don't wait for divine intervention. Let every member of the family have a hand in organizing their own space.

- Do something nice for yourself. Instead of overeating in response to stress, take a long bath, settle down with a favorite book, watch a funny movie, get a massage or facial (yes, men, you too!), or write in your daily journal. All are guaranteed to keep you out of the fridge and engaged in your new healthy lifestyle.

Mouth

- Reconsider your coping strategies. Under stress, women and children tend to run to food (carb and fat combos) and men to alcohol. Heads up to all of you: Neither constitutes good stress management. There are better ways to learn to calm down.

- Did you realize that *stressed* spelled backward is *desserts*? There's solid science to show that stress can lead you to overeat carbs and fat. Make a plan to thwart overeating due to stress. For the next 24 hours, take note of your overeating triggers, as well as the time of day they tend to occur. Anything could trigger overeating, so keep an open mind.

- Plan for the tough times. Mid-afternoon is one of the hardest in terms of susceptibility to overeating, especially for women. Make sure you have stress-neutralizing foods on hand. Excellent sources of protein are low-fat cheese, yogurt, chicken soup, cottage cheese, a protein shake, or an energy bar. Excellent sources of carbohydrates include whole-grain crackers, whole-wheat pita, fruits, and veggies. Healthy fats like nut butters and olives also help nix stress-overdrive cravings.

Muscle

- Engaging in physical activity is a particularly helpful way to neutralize stress. The next time you feel that "fight-or flight" reaction going into high gear, get up and move. *Do not* walk over to the vending machine! Just fire up a nice five- to ten-minute walk or go out and shoot some hoops and note how you feel afterward. You should have a great sense of calmness and control. As a bonus, physical activity helps to control your appetite.

- Try a walking meditation. Practitioners of yoga have been doing this for stress relief and centering for centuries. Just find a peaceful place to walk, clear your head of troubles, allow your mind to be calm, and concentrate on your serene surroundings. You're secreting healing beta endorphins to calm you at the same time you're getting in more physical activity.

It's a Generational Thing

Kids 7–12

Mind

- I bet you figured out that it's hard to take care of yourself when you have loads of homework and are trying to keep up with after-school activities and friends. Don't freak out over this. You're learning how to balance eating well, getting good sleep, staying active, and having fun. Get Mom and Dad to help you learn how to figure out what's most important to do first.

- Don't be afraid to talk to a family member or friend when you feel worried and sad. There are times in life when it's really important to get that loving support. Start to do this now at your young age, and it will become one of your most valuable stress-busting tools as you grow older.

Mouth

- Ever notice that when you're upset you feel like eating, especially sweet foods? Well, it turns out that it happens to lots of people. Make sure you're eating a healthy after-school snack, and if you still feel like chewing, then try sugar-free gum or a small piece of crunchy fruit like an apple. Stay away from the sugary stuff. It's trouble.

Muscle

- Here's something new to try when you feel like busting out of your skin with anxiety and stress—hop on your bike and keep on peddlin'. You probably didn't know that when you get up and do something active like that, you help yourself to feel better. And afterwards you're more able to get your homework and house chores done instead of feeling hopeless about them.

Teens 13–19

Mind

• Cramming for exams can stress you out. The last thing on your mind is eating right and being active. Instead of becoming a hurricane of anxiety, prevent problems by learning how to prioritize your time. It's all about balancing your life's work with self-care. Your teen years are a great time to start practicing this.

Mouth

• Come on now, it's your third week and your challenge is to attack your funky eating habits with small steps. So here are some options: Eat a simple and healthy breakfast the majority of mornings; steer clear of vending machines; avoid fried foods and pizza in the cafeteria; choose healthy option like grilled chicken wraps at the fast food place; limit yourself to diet sodas and to no more than two a day.

Muscle

• While guys are more likely to do something active, teen girls want to hang out and talk. So, girls, this is a special heads up to you: Get your friends together and hit the gym or dance class as a group. It's fun. You can talk while you're on the treadmills or hang out after class, and at the same time you can encourage one another. Try to spend time with kids who think like you and are more active and enjoy moving their bodies.

20s

Mind

• Make the mind-body connection. Learn how to be mindful about when and what you eat. When you exercise, pay attention to how your body feels.

• Even though you're young and energetic, try to remember to get in *at least* six hours of sleep so that you can wake up refreshed and on track with your self-care and better able to deal with the day's stresses.

Mouth

• You are the dashboard dining generation. Yep, you're the grab-and-go champs. If you must do it, at least choose better foods. Warm a whole-wheat pita in the microwave, stuff it with two or three slices of low-fat cheese, and then zap it for a few seconds more to melt it. With this and an apple, you now have a 60-second snack that's balanced and contains whole foods. This is about customizing your crazy on-the-run lifestyle with healthy eating.

Muscle

• Join the company softball, soccer, or volleyball team. Heck, it's just for fun. It's a great way to meet new people, use your body, and release the stresses of work.

30s

Mind

• Thirty-year-olds who juggle family, work, and community obligations have written the book on stress. This is the key time to maintain your self-care, but keep it simple. Make a plan and schedule times to walk, hit the gym, or see a friend. That's right. You have to schedule these things or they won't happen.

• Learn stress-management skills, and start to practice them this week. In your journal, record how you were able to face down a life stressor without overeating or engaging in any kind of self-destructive behaviors like smoking, drinking, getting angry, or withdrawing.

• You may be stressing out over the health of your family. Never nag. You'll be most successful when they see you setting an example and getting results.

Mouth

- Avoid wingin' it through the day. You know what I mean. Defend your right to eat well, and be assertive about making the time to shop for and prepare healthy foods. This is the way you honor your body. Nourishing it healthfully during your 30s is fundamental to achieving and maintaining your wellness. If you can do it now, you can do it much more easily as you age.

Muscle

- Get out that stroller and walk or run with the little one. If you don't have kids, then it's all about ritualizing your physical activity routine. It's important to experiment with what works for you in terms of what, where, and when you do it. If you're schedule crazy, learn to be flexible. But do get it done.

40s

Mind

- The 40s have the potential for significant stressors: medical conditions, job changes, relationships that come and go, kids reappearing with crises, and parents aging and needing care. This is the prime time to hone those regrouping skills and practice mental flexibility. Learn how to navigate between Plan A and Plan B, or up to Z! Master regroupers can get and keep the optimal level of wellness and health.

- Learn "relaxation response" meditation and practice it at least once a day. The idea is to sit quietly and consciously relax each muscle group in your body, starting from your toes and working up to your face, while breathing deeply and evenly.

- You need seven to eight hours sleep a day, minimum, to maintain optimal immune function, to feel energized for your morning workout, and to be alert and mindful about how and what to eat.

Mouth

- Many people in their 40s work long hours as their careers peak, and it's easy to skip lunches or mindlessly eat take-out at work while tapping away at the computer. BYOF: Bring Your Own Food. For snacks, keep fresh fruit at the office, along with yogurt, cottage cheese, pre-made protein shakes, low-fat peanut butter, and whole-wheat crackers. If you don't bring lunch, then choose user-friendly delis and restaurants with plenty of whole-food options.

Muscle

• Feeling a difference in your strength and endurance? The third week is when you can start to see changes that motivate you to continue the Challenge. Next time you lift weights or take that walk, put a little more energy into your workout. You're ready to ramp it up. Celebrate your increasing fitness. Way to go!

50s

Mind

• Getting through this third week is a grand achievement. So many people in their 50s give up if they don't see radical changes overnight. Don't go there. Be patient and persistent. Practice my replace the "but" with the "and" exercise. Instead of saying, "I've removed six pounds in three weeks, *but* I have so far to go," say "I've removed six pounds in three weeks, *and* I am so proud of myself, *and* I will continue to work at this." One is defeatist and the other is proactive and positive. It's amazing what one little word can do!

Mouth

• There *is* life after having a smaller dinner! Instead of saving all of your calories for a big meal, spread them out throughout the day by eating every three to four hours. When you do, your dinners are lighter and you're less apt to gain weight. As you age, the rule is that dinners get lighter but are still satisfying. Load up on vegetables to accompany your protein, and go light on the starches.

Muscle

• Thirty-minute power naps can be helpful during the day when stress interrupts your nighttime sleep schedule. When you do this, you're more likely to have the energy to keep your physical activity going.

• Be patient with yourself. You won't rebound to an active lifestyle overnight. Your goal is 80 percent compliance with eating and exercise.

60s and Beyond

Mind

• Many of your stressors now are about disabilities, care giving, medical conditions, and finances. Don't let them erode your wonderful wellness goals. Overstressing, ruminating, and being anxious all the time ages you rapidly. It interferes with memory, learning, and moods. Instead, adopt a little wit and humor; step back and really look at where your priorities are. You'll then see that most of your stressors aren't that important. It's all about being healthy and happy enough to enjoy the real priorities: your family and loved ones.

Mouth

• You may think that your eating habits are set; just like you think you're generally set in your ways. Not true. There's still plenty of time to be adventuresome in a healthy way. Color up your diet with new fruits and vegetables, ways to eat (more vegetarian?), recipes, and restaurants. As you age, it's important to keep your eating a dynamic process. It's all about nourishing an aging body that wants to maintain optimal vigor and vitality.

Muscle

• Check out your neighborhood and community for innovative and fun senior physical activities. Today there are trainers who specialize in helping people over 60 get and stay physically strong and independent.

• It's imperative that you start doing balance exercises. This includes the use of balance boards as well as balance-focused movement techniques such as Feldenkrais (a way of working with the awareness of one's body to improve movement and enhance human functioning). You need help to do this, so go to the senior center or find a trainer and get the appropriate instruction. After 60, strength, endurance, and flexibility are joined by balance as essential components of optimal physical fitness.

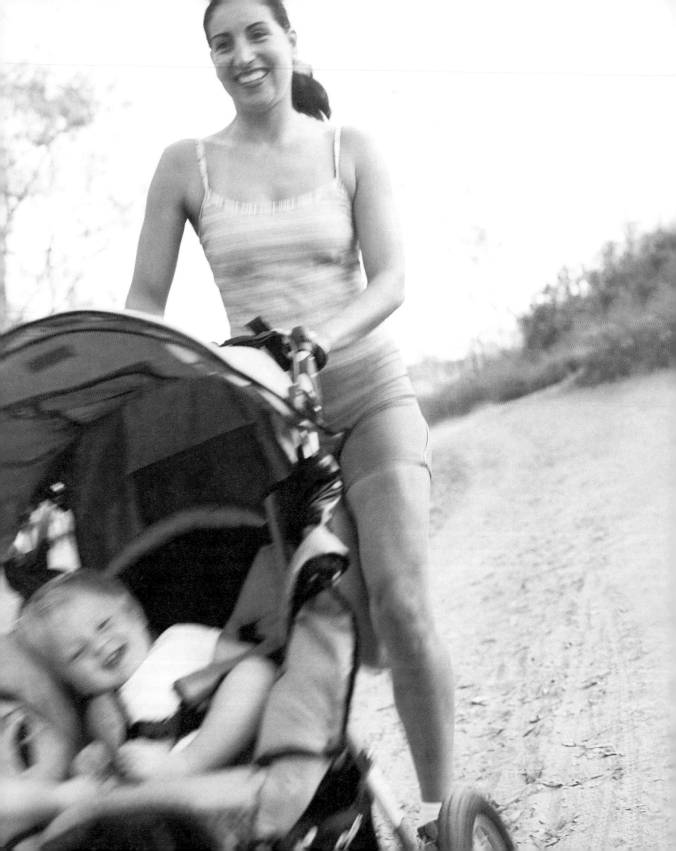

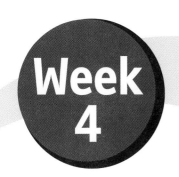

Being a
Road
Warrior

Sure, it would be easier to stay on the program if you were home all day and in complete control of your time. But that just doesn't apply to most of us. When you're commuting, ferrying the kids from activity to activity, or taking business trips, you can still stick with the National Body Challenge—all it takes is a little planning.

Take it on the road! Road warriors—that is, anyone who lives in the car (salespeople, soccer moms and dads, kids with a heavy after-school activity schedules)—need to maintain a healthy lifestyle while out and about. Same applies when you're traveling longer distances for work or pleasure.

Week 4 Rules and Tools

Mind

• Regroup for the road. Make a Plan T for travel. Pack a cooler with healthy food if you're carpooling for hours or stuck at after-school activities. Roll up your sweats and sneakers when you leave town on business. It's all about learning how to shift from Plan A (home) to Plan T (travelin'). People who do this well look, feel, and live like it.

• Stay out of that hotel mini-bar. You know who you are! You're pooped, and that candy is calling to you. Don't even accept the mini-bar key when you check in. That way you can avoid this temptation.

Mouth

• Learn about healthy snacks. For the right combination of high-quality protein, fat, and carbs, pack an energy bar (containing 10–20 grams of protein, 10–30 grams of carbohydrates, and 2–6 grams of fat with no more than 3 grams of saturated fat), or mix together unsalted nuts and dried fruit like raisins, cherries, or apples. One palm-full of this mixture is a serving.

• Know your fast-food eateries—many now offer healthier menu items. Try grilled fish, chicken salad, or a grilled chicken sandwich (hold the mayo) for lunch or dinner. Be sure you know which selections are health-friendly. Many restaurants keep nutritional breakdowns on the premises; you only have to ask for them. Or go to the companies' Websites to find the info and know what to order before you even go in.

• Watch out for coffee shops. Grabbing a cup of coffee with skim milk is fine, but steer clear of the pastries. Still really want something sweet—without consuming a ton of calories? Go for biscotti instead of muffins, cookies, or scones. They are the least likely to get you into trouble.

- Plane and train warriors need even more planning. Start the day with a great breakfast. This means protein (eggs, yogurt, milk, cottage cheese, low-fat cheese, a breakfast patty, a protein shake) and whole grains (oatmeal, whole-wheat toast, high-fiber cereal), along with healthy fat (walnuts, almonds).

- Stay hydrated. While traveling, you need to be aware of your water needs. Don't wait until you're dry as a desert, panting for water. On hot days, especially, plan on having a 12–16 oz. bottle of water with you all the time, and drink no less than three to four bottles a day.

- I realize that it's hard to manage your eating when you can't completely control your schedule, but try to avoid late-night snacking—it's the easiest way to gain weight. If you can't avoid it, opt for lighter fare when eating after 8 P.M. In any event, try to stick to eating at least every three to four hours to quell your appetite and spread the calories throughout the day.

- Eat out wisely. Have just one piece of whole-grain bread at lunch and none for dinner. Fill up on water, non-creamy soup, and salad before having your entree. Eat no more than a deck of cards–size piece of meat or fish. Take the rest home. Order your salad with dressing on the side. Twist your fork in the dressing and then drizzle it onto the greens to get optimal taste with minimal calories. Also, substitute additional vegetables for pasta or rice when ordering your entree. Share dessert.

Muscle

- Get in your physical activity. Be sure to pack your sneakers and work-out clothes. Try to patronize hotels that have health-club facilities. If they don't, ask if they offer a guest pass to a local gym. And if that fails, get out and walk. While traveling, it's important to get in at least 15–30 minutes of cardio daily to keep yourself mentally and physically fresh and strong. It will also help you sleep better in a different time zone.

- Do you find yourself at your kid's game or practice for hours on end? Don't just sit there! Bring your sneakers, and use this opportunity to get up and clock some steps on your pedometer!

It's a Generational Thing

Kids 7–12

Mind

- Ever wonder what Mom and Dad do when they have to be away from home and still want to eat right and exercise? Well, it's not easy. Ask them about it. Let them teach you how you have to think ahead to get it done. Never forget that your best teachers are your parents. They love you and want the best for you. Plus, this gives you some precious time to hang out with them. All right, they're grownups and all. But they're yours, and that's special.

Mouth

- Your parents are going to make sure you have healthy foods and snacks available when you're away from home at school games or while driving to visit relatives or going on vacation. Help your mom and dad choose delicious and healthy foods that you like for road trips. Remember, you have a say in this. It's your tummy!

Muscle

- When you go on vacation this year, leave the video games at home. Beaches are meant for walking and playing on, mountains are there to climb and explore, and lakes and oceans are for swimming in. Take advantage of them to have fun and get healthy.

Teens 13–19

Mind

- There are many opportunities in a teen's life when you'll be away from home: camp, studying abroad, and visiting out-of-state friends and family. Staying on your wellness program isn't easy when you're surrounded by so much temptation. Cheap, low-quality foods are everywhere. Don't let this get to you. Instead, be strong and focused on looking and feeling great, not mindlessly letting it all go.

Mouth

- Want to treat yourself to, say, a special dessert while on the road? No problem. All you have to do is realize that all foods come with a price. It just depends on what you're willing to pay. I'd recommend the economy option, which means sharing your treat, eating it slowly, and savoring it. This is all about learning the fine art of tasting. People who taste, don't wear their food the next morning. The price is right!

Muscle

- Do you think that just because you're on the road all bets are off when it comes to physical activity? Think again. Bet yourself (a nonfood reward) that you can get in at least a walk every day you're away. *I* bet you can! More important, if you're visiting someone who totally gets it with staying active, ask to join him or her at their club or outdoor activity.

20s

Mind

- This is a mobile society, and you're no exception. You have the freedom to visit distant friends at the drop of a hat or travel to exotic locations for some R & R. Arm yourself with a healthy, realistic attitude before you go. Know that you'll probably be eating and drinking differently. That's okay. Just stay active and keep the balance going so that there's no weight gain. Achieving that balance during your youthful road warrior days is a marvelous accomplishment.

Mouth

- These are the party years, so watch the alcohol. The more you drink, the more uninhibited you become, which means that you stop paying attention to what you eat. Avoid hard liquor because of the calories, and limit yourself to no more than two beers or glasses of wine.

Muscle

- Jump rope—it's a great portable cardio workout that you can do anywhere. Ever wonder why boxers do this to train? It's a challenge to keep that jumping going minute after minute. Start out slowly and build up to 60-second intervals of jumping, for five sets. It's great for the heart, and keeps you focused on your coordination and agility.

30s

Mind

• Take the whole family on adventures. Share activities that keep kids and parents moving and fit. Learn to integrate this kind of thinking into vacations and weekend outings. Teach your children that a healthy lifestyle is a vital part of living, whether you're at home or on the road.

Mouth

• The family car is a great venue for healthy eating since you're in control. Pack sandwiches made with multigrain bread, fresh lettuce, tomatoes, and turkey or chicken. Yogurt with sliced almonds, cottage cheese, low-fat cheese sticks, and hard-boiled eggs all work as snacks and mini meals.

• If you've had a wonderful day of recreational activities and have burned loads of calories, go ahead and enjoy that good meal! Keep your portions small and eat slowly. Share a dessert. Just remember to enjoy each bite.

Muscle

• If you're kept busy with kids, recognize that this may be one of the hardest times in your life to get some physical activity in, so aim for balance. Keep telling yourself that the best caregiver is a healthy caregiver. Your loved ones are depending on you to be there for them. You can't do that if you're under par physically, which makes you feel bad mentally. Avoid that vicious cycle and just do what you can given your time constraints. Little steps keep your metabolic fires going. When you do have more time, go for it.

• For you busy moms, learn how to feel more comfortable about delegating child care and chores to others. You have to be assertive about finding time to get out and walk or take that class. You need this to help you stem the tide of stress and keep sane. And this is especially true when you're on the road.

40s

Mind

• Nearly everyone in their 40s is traveling more. Business travel is rampant. There are grown children as well as grandchildren to visit. Or, you've been saving up for that cruise or special vacation. If you're traveling for any reason, keep a persistent mental attitude by taking your healthy living habits on the road.

Mouth

• Stay hydrated with water as well as with healthy fruits and veggies. Yep, they're packed with water and nutritious vitamins and minerals. The sugars are healthy fructose and can help keep you energized throughout your busy day. They're the best snack to carry around.

Muscle

• Break up your workouts into smaller time increments, and add them up at the end of a busy day.

• If you're doing the road-warrior thing, buy a resistance tubing set and take it with you. You'll be able to do strength and flexibility workouts in your hotel room or anywhere you want. Have someone show you how to use the tubing correctly so you can get the maximum benefit from your workout. Combine this with your daily cardio program.

50s

Mind

• Many people in their 50s can't wait to travel. In addition to business, there's so much interest in seeing other cultures. Unfortunately, a lot of you haven't kept up with your wellness programs and are now feeling less able to stay independent and enjoy traveling. Not to worry. Anyone can turn this around by focusing on health and changing poor lifestyle choices. Your Target Motivation could be to be able to travel anywhere you want to; and embrace each day with vim, vigor, and vitality.

Mouth

• When out and about and tempted to try new foods, learn the art of sharing—and for you that means entrees. Most restaurant portions are mountainous, and who needs all that food? Instead, how about ordering two appetizers and a salad? Or having a salad and splitting the entree? Save the calories for a shared dessert as a treat. And remember to "pay" for any treat with your daily physical activity.

Muscle

• How about planning an adventure vacation? Many travel tour operators offer great hiking, biking, rafting, and sightseeing trips in the U.S. and overseas for people 50 years and older. Come on, push your envelope!

60s and Beyond

Mind

• Develop a "can do" attitude. "Sure I can hike that trail, make the summit, and enjoy the panorama." Those of you in your 60s and beyond who believe they can get up and embrace each day always seem to achieve that goal. Think of the wonderful places you can visit and people you will meet, because you *can*. And for you parents and grandparents out there, remember that you're teachers. Your family is looking to you to be an example that, no matter what your age, you can still be healthy.

Mouth

• Try new ethnic foods, test your palate, and open your mind to fresh culinary experiences. Don't be shy. Men, try some soy. It's a great source of protein. Women, increase your intake of fish for those valuable omega-3 fatty acids. Wherever you visit, ask and learn about new foods. This is part of the total enjoyment of nourishing your body and your spirit.

Muscle

- While traveling, support one another in your quest to stay fit. Sign up for hikes, bike rides, and walking adventures together. Or if you're single—heck, why not make new friends by joining outdoor activities, as well as travel clubs with like-minded individuals. You have to get in that cardio every day you can and keep strong with your weights so that you can even participate. The reward is so worth the work you're doing to stay fit.

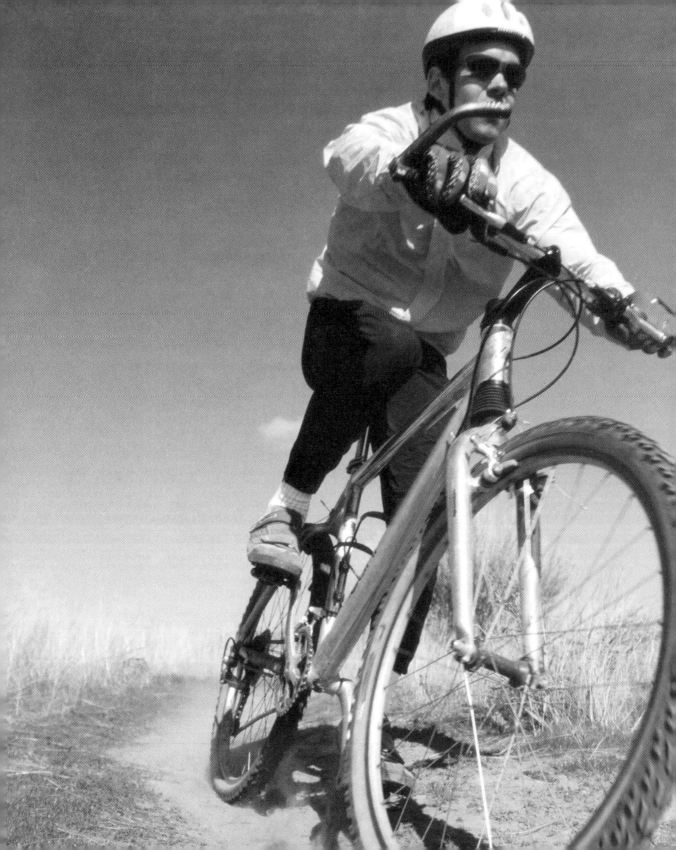

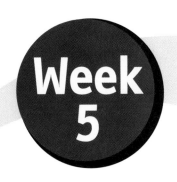

Week 5

Fine-Tuning
Your Program

If you've decided to do the 8-week program, you're now at the halfway point. You now have two options. If you're taking the 12-week Challenge, you're a third of the way through. Whatever the case, you're a winner. You'll take the lessons you've learned and keep practicing, honing, and refining them for the rest of your life.

135

You'll pick up this book and revisit it endless times to refresh your memory about the rules and tools. And, you can keep rechallenging yourself with another 8- or 12-week program. Remember, this is a lifelong journey.

If you've been consistent, you're seeing results. Your body composition is changing as you're removing fat and training your muscles. Let's do some updating and some tweaking of your program to keep the results coming. After all, we don't want to get stuck in a plateau! Stay alert!

Week 5 Rules and Tools

Mind

- Now is a great time to grab your National Body Challenge contract and read it aloud to yourself. How are you doing? Look at those Mind, Mouth, and Muscle goals you wrote down that first week. Identify specific challenges, and redo your goals in each category. For instance, if eating breakfast is no longer an issue, then write down what is: staying up too late and munching mountains in front of the TV?

- Slip on your "clothes-o-meter." Well? If it's getting looser—and maybe actually fits by now—congratulations!

- Get out that Target Motivation. Is it still effective? Do you need a new one? If so, go back to Chapter 2 and redo the Target Motivation exercise. Otherwise, it's onward and upward!

Mouth

- Ramp up your level of mindfulness. After all, it was mindlessness that got you in this mess in the first place. Time how long it takes you to eat a meal. Then next day, take twice as long. Chewing every bite carefully, you'll experiencing the texture and flavor (and eat less).

- Beware of buffets. They're especially difficult for people who just don't know when to say "when." Use a smaller plate to limit yourself, and only belly up to the table once instead of making repeat trips. Try small servings of lots of interesting foods.

- Watch your portions. Hey, you may be eating your designated meals and snacks, but if you're packing away mountains of food at each sitting, that will stall your weight-loss efforts. A calorie is a calorie even when it comes from healthy foods. Revisit the calorie calculator in Chapter 2, and make sure you're eating the right amount.

• Don't trust restaurant serving sizes. Remember that we live in a "super-size" world. Look at the plate in front of you and divide the rice, pasta, or potato portion by a third to half. Eat one portion and leave the rest.

• Be aware of the bloat factor. Some men and women are salt-sensitive and bloat from it. Starches tend to bloat women. When in doubt, spend a day or two eliminating as much salt and starch as possible from your diet, and check your bloat as well as your weight.

Muscle

• Reassess your cardio workouts. Make sure you're doing some at least five times a week, and intensify your sessions by increasing speed and/or difficulty with more resistance (a hill).

• Remember, if you don't lift weight, you don't remove weight. If you've been going great with cardio but doing little or no weight lifting, a plateau is a friendly reminder that you absolutely must do some form of resistance training twice a week to maintain an optimally hot metabolism and keep the weight loss happening.

It's a Generational Thing

Kids 7–12

Mind

• Give yourself a high five! This is your fifth week, and you've been hanging in there, slugging it out with the family as you all participate in the National Body Challenge. This week is special because it's a time to check out how you've been doing all along and refine things a bit. Take out those clothes you love and see how they fit now.

Mouth

• Do you notice that you've gotten used to eating better? Name three things you've done to improve your eating habits. Are there even more? Tell your mom or dad which new foods you've tried and liked that replace junk food from the past. You see? You've done well! Now, make a list of the next three habits you want to change in your eating. How about trying not to eat junk food at your friends' homes? Think you can do that? How about eating one portion of food at meals instead of two or three? I *know* you can do that!

Muscle

• Instead of asking for video games or movies on DVD as birthday or holiday presents this year, ask for a bike, roller blades, a soccer ball, dance lessons, or sports equipment instead.

Teens 13–19

Mind

• Don't discount any changes you've made as being "too small." Everything counts. Adjust your expectations, and make realistic goals. After putting on your "clothes-o-meter," congratulate yourself for a job well done, and then get serious about rampin' it up a bit to meet your overall goal. So take a deep breath, and let's reenergize now.

Mouth

• Do you ever feel that you're fooling yourself by saying that you're eating well when you're really not? This week get honest with yourself about those extra snacks, portion sizes, and late-night eating habits that are still happening. Then commit to substituting fruits, vegetables, and whole grains for any junk you're still eating, day or night. Swear off refined sugar whenever you can, especially those soft drinks.

Muscle

• Make physical activity more fun. How about dancing? For that matter, what about dance lessons? Most gyms and community centers have wonderful dance classes—jazz, tap, hip-hop, whatever you want. Plug into your MP3 player or iPod and dance away. You can easily toast 300 calories with 30 to 45 minutes of hard-core dancing.

20s

Mind

• Look at where you can improve. What are your vulnerable points? Lack of consistency, larger-than-necessary portions, poor planning, scheduling, and emotional issues are all things to consider. Work on these tough challenges now.

Mouth

• Clean up your eating by reading food labels. Cut down on or eliminate those foods that contain high-fructose corn syrup, hydrogenated or partially hydrogenated oils, and trans fats that are common in processed junk food.

Muscle

• Go all the way, and participate in a sports event. Try your first 5K walk or run. That goal will keep you focused and bring it all together.

30s

Mind

• As you review your original National Body Challenge goals, remind yourself that this decade is often the most hectic and challenging. Cut yourself some slack, and realize that every small step is actually a huge accomplishment; given how busy you are. Whether you're a single man or woman, a childless couple, or have chosen to start a family, the 30s are a tough time. Acknowledge your efforts thus far, and simply build on them for the rest of your Challenge—and beyond.

• Sleep is a gift at this age as people tug at you from all directions. Use soothing music, baths, a book, meditation—anything you can find to help improve the quality of your sleep.

Mouth

• Quit multitasking while you're eating. More mindless calories are consumed by people stuffing their faces while pounding away on computer keyboards, talking on the phone, or driving! Try not to do five things while you're eating. Get the TV out of the kitchen, let the phone take messages, and sit down and enjoy your meal.

Muscle

• Find a new place to work out. There are alternatives to the classic gym setting. It could be a yoga or dance studio. Try for a place that has good child care if you have little ones. Start looking today.

40s

Mind

• During your 40s there's a greater chance to be blindsided by divorce, job changes, illnesses, or physical disabilities. Turn any of these into an opportunity to rise to the occasion and practice your regrouping skills. The 40s are all about refining these skills as new problems surface seemingly every day. Stay focused. Polish up that Target Motivation, and use it every day to help guide you.

Mouth

• If you've reached a plateau or feel as if the weight removal is too slow despite excellent compliance with the physical activity, take a moment and thoroughly assess your eating habits. If you haven't been good about keeping your food journals, start today. You need the data to see what's going on. Look again at quality, quantity, and frequency in your eating habits. A common mistake is eating high-quality foods in excessive portions. The good news is that it's healthy food. Unfortunately, it's mountains of healthy food. Or perhaps you've gotten careless about having that mid-afternoon snack, so essential to controlling your dinner portions. Whatever it is, regroup and focus on your problem areas.

Muscle

• It's time to do more activities of daily living. How about the garage or closet from hell that you've sworn to clean for the last ten years? Okay, today's the day. That means burning lots of calories mentally and physically as you figure out what to toss and what to keep. You'll be scrubbing and repainting and reorganizing. It all sounds like a superb use of time and muscle power!

50s

Mind

• As you reassess your progress this week, connect the dots on the relationship between lifestyle and medical conditions. Are you doing everything you can to optimize your opportunities to practicing healthy living? Being more aware of how your eating and physical-activity behavior allows you to be more stress resilient and calm. This, in turn, strengthens your immune system and allows you to reduce the risk of diseases like cancer.

Mouth

• Here's a nifty trick to help keep those dinner portions under control. Make a shake in the mid-afternoon. You'll find out how on page 51. It's a healthy, delicious and very satisfying snack that will put a serious dent in dinner appetites.

Muscle

• Do you have a particularly stressful event or activity you must participate in? Nothing calms you down better than a little physical activity before you undergo stress—public speaking, taking a test, or confronting a work colleague. So, use your innate body chemicals (endorphins, serotonin) to help you stay focused and centered. Physical activity is not just about buffed bodies. It's really about buffed minds as well!

60s and Beyond

Mind

• As you look at your original goals and objectives, you may realize that you've made enough progress in four weeks to affect some of the medical conditions you may have. Have your blood pressure, blood sugar, or cholesterol levels checked. If you've been consistent on the National Body Challenge, you're guaranteed to have positively impacted these conditions. Mentally, this has to be so gratifying. Make sure you're pacing this with your primary-care providers so that they know how to make adjustments in your medications and when to do further assessments. Keep the momentum going!

Mouth

• As you reassess the progress you've made over the past four weeks, check how you're doing in eliminating processed foods from your diet. This is so important, as science has clearly shown that continually eating these foods is detrimental to your health. Strive to eat mostly whole foods.

• Keep yourself well hydrated throughout the day. Plunk some sliced lemons or oranges into a pitcher of water and drink up all day long.

Muscle

• Studies have shown that all of us, especially women, are very concerned about losing their physical independence after 50. Women want to continue to caregive to others, and men want to be able to drive and walk and enjoy life as long as they can. Well, you can't do any of this without the strength to get out of a chair (that's a squat in weight lifting) or walking (endurance). Also, nothing is more important than preventing a fall, and if you do fall, preventing a fracture and surgery. The best prevention is to maintain endurance, strength, flexibility, and balance. The best reward for your consistency with the National Body Challenge is lifelong independence, both mentally and physically.

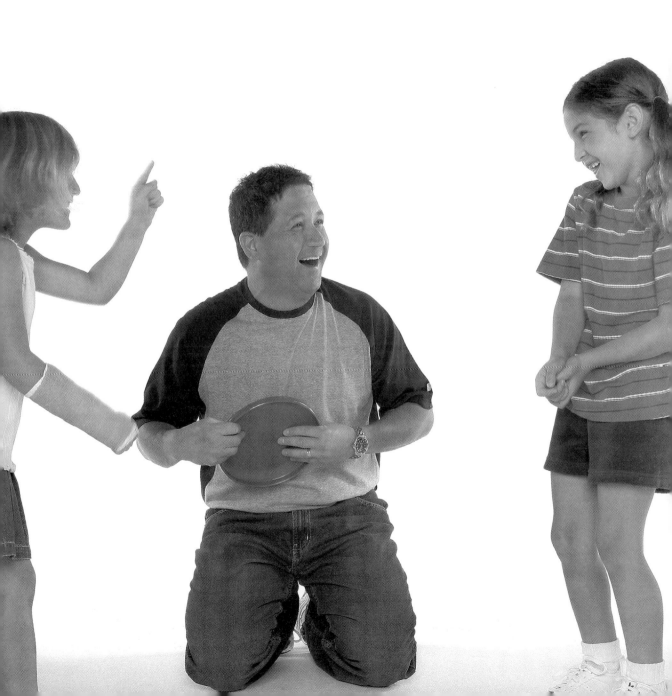

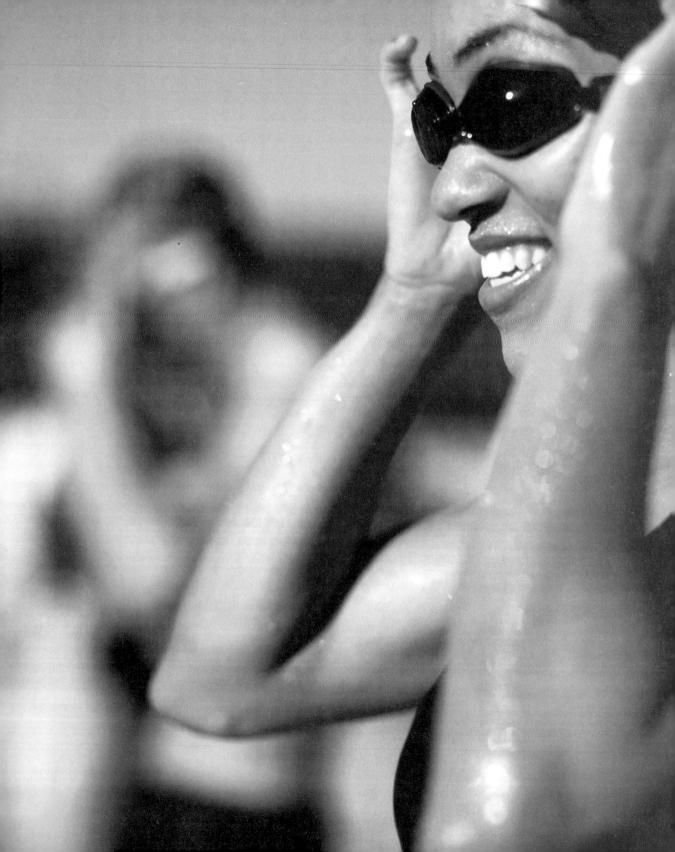

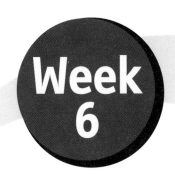

Keeping
Your
Commitment

This week can be a danger zone for a number of reasons. You're looking good now, people are starting to comment, and you might become a little careless about sticking to the regimen. The biggest myth is that once you reach a particular goal you can relax and coast. Wrong! The truth is that you have to keep on keepin' on. Work it every single day.

The good news is that through practice, it gets easier, and eventually you don't really think much about it because it's become a way of life.

Another reason that this week is potentially a danger zone is that strange relationship issues surface once you start seeing changes. Just when you think that everyone is happy for your success and progress, friends and family members pull back and might actually sabotage you. What's that about? Well, your success is causing them to reflect on their own lives. If they're not working toward a healthy lifestyle, too, then your success can be threatening and intimidating. The key is to be open and honest and to communicate your true feelings. Don't preach or police; just be open to discussion and then get on with your own healthy behaviors.

You are a living inspiration for people who are ready to change. For everyone else, just carry on and let them discover their journey when it's right for them. And, pay attention to any vulnerable times you might slip up. Onward and upward!

Week 6 Rules and Tools

Mind

- Don't give up if you slip. Embrace tough days as times to learn how to face up to a challenge and work around it. Expect obstacles to happen, and practice regrouping each time. Remember, mistakes are opportunities to learn, and to build a strong foundation for healthy living.

- What if your partner, family member, or friend seems to be sabotaging your efforts? It's time for a sit-down. You need to be straightforward about your perceptions of their behavior. Let them know that you're committed to achieving your goal and will not be dissuaded by their negative efforts. Try to get them to talk about their own feelings of potential threat and/or intimidation by your success. Please understand that your success may make people reflect on their own lives, and that can be quite uncomfortable.

- Practice stress resilience if your spouse or partner tries to sabotage your efforts. Work around them. If he or she insists upon bringing sweets into the house, practice saying "No, thank you" and sticking to your guns. Do not be dissuaded!

- Cut yourself some slack. During eight weeks, life happens. If an event, trip, injury, or persuasive partner derails you for a bit, don't beat yourself up. Simply hop back on the train when you can and continue your National Body Challenge journey.

Mouth

• Don't get careless just because your "clothes-o-meter" is actually fitting you. Get a new one, the next size down, to keep you honest. When you go to that party or function, avoid wearing loose clothing. Snug-fitting clothes make you more aware of your eating.

• Manage celebrations. Learn how to enjoy yourself without going overboard and regretting it the next day. Before attending a special event where food will be served, do your daily exercise. That's like putting money in the bank because it frees up some calories to spend on food.

• Deal with dessert. Have a piece of birthday cake or a serving of luscious dessert, but eat it slowly and savor the experience. Put your fork down at least three times and take 10 breaths between bites. Learn to share. The more the merrier. If you end up eating only a third of that chocolate mousse, well done. It will save you the fat and calories, as well as teaching you, once again, how to savor.

• Call ahead. If you know the hostess or host of the event, tell her or him that you don't eat red meat or ask if there will be a choice of fruit for dessert rather than the pie. Most people are more than happy to accommodate their guests' needs. Offer to bring a dish of veggies, fruit, or healthy protein to share with others.

• Watch the alcohol. People often think that a special occasion gives them license to drink to excess. Alcohol makes it difficult to make wise food choices, packs on lots of calories, and is just plain dangerous to your progress. Your best choice is a wine spritzer (half a glass of wine mixed with soda water). It's refreshing, and half the calories of straight wine.

Muscle

• Regroup around injuries. Try not to get frustrated. Avoid the tendency to do no exercise if you can't do the sport you love because you're hurt. Show your stress resilience and work around it. If you can't walk or run, then now is a great time to ramp up your weight training and perfect your form, do core work, and perhaps hop in the pool. Everyone experiences some kind of problem along the path to fitness. Be creative if you've injured a knee, an ankle, or a hip. Work with what you do have.

- Don't forget to make it fun. The more enjoyment you're getting from your physical activity, the more you'll want to get right back to it. It's all about increasing the joy of having a healthy, fit body.

It's a Generational Thing

Kids 7–12

Mind

- Do you realize that this is your sixth week of the National Body Challenge? Make a list of the changes in your body that you've noticed. Has your family noticed as well? How about your friends and other kids? This is all about learning that persistence pays off. If you want to achieve anything in life, you have to hang in there and work at it. And do this without doing everything perfectly or stressing out too much about it. Remember, for kids it really is a team effort with the whole family. When you win, everyone wins! Keep up that positive attitude now!

Mouth

- What do you do when you go to a friend's house or a party or you're at school and you're tempted by all the goodies? Well, by now you've discovered that you can indeed have some treats. It's all about eating more slowly and having one portion. You don't have to feel deprived at all. You have the best of all worlds. You're balancing your healthy eating with treats here and there. Well done!

Muscle

- Try to avoid just sitting around playing a video game or staring at the TV. For that matter, make it a habit to watch no more than one hour of TV per school day and use the extra time playing outside with friends.

Teens 13–19

Mind

• The teen years are so tough psychologically as you're maturing into a new stage of life. The carefree days of childhood are now a thing of the past. You often become more self-conscious about appearance, and suddenly sexuality is a big deal. Both girls and boys can be troubled by a shaky sense of self-esteem and self-worth. Peer pressure is on. This is also the time that eating disorders start showing up, especially in you girls, as you take drastic measures to fit in—literally, into those size-zero jeans. This transition can be challenging.

    Make a point this week to talk it out with your parents or, if that's impossible, a trusted family member or friend. It's so important to put these body changes into perspective. Share any feelings of insecurity you have, and listen to the wise words of someone who knows you well and wants to help guide you to a renewed sense of happiness.

Mouth

• If you've been doing well, parents and friends may make the mistake of saying, "Hey, you look great, so stop trying so hard now" and offer you foods you should be avoiding. It's usually well intended, but delivers the wrong message—that the work is over. It's never over; it just gets easier. So politely tell them, "Thanks but no thanks," and stay with your National Body Challenge program.

• If you're having problems sticking with the program because you're having emotional problems resulting in stress overeating or even undereating, you really need to get help. Tell your parents, and get an appointment with a professional who can help guide you through this tough time.

Muscle

• Let's get it straight. The sexiest body is a fit-looking one. That's true for both boys and girls. You don't get that way by sitting around. You also don't achieve that goal through dietary changes alone. You need the whole package—a stress-resilient mind, good nutrition, and physical fitness. Make it a habit to go to the gym with friends, join a soccer or softball team for fun, and don't forget volunteer work that keeps you up and movin' (think Habitat for Humanity).

20s

Mind

• As you think of connecting with potential life partners, remember that your success in keeping fit and healthy will be greatly influenced by your choices. Veer toward like-minded folks who embrace a healthy lifestyle and you'll have a built-in support system that's constantly encouraging you to stay on track and strengthen your commitment to healthy living.

Mouth

• You may be running around doing the 20-something lifestyle, but by Week 6 you've probably noted that your eating habits have really changed—nothing radical, just enough to make a difference in your energy and appearance. Don't stop now; you're on a roll. Reassess, and find at least two more things you can do to continue to refine your eating behavior. Still succumbing to that high-calorie coffee drink every day? All 500 calories with 20 grams of fat and 40 grams of refined sugar? Have a skim-milk latte instead. Go lean and mean!

Muscle

• Are you still having a bear of a time trying to wedge some physical activity into your work and social calendar? Well, by Week 6 you've had lots of time to learn to be creative and make it happen. It's time to really bite the bullet. Stuff your workout clothes into a duffel bag and throw it into your car. Recommit to going after work, and just plain do it. Don't ruminate.

30s

Mind

• If you have a family, then by now you should have established new daily lifestyle patterns. Take a moment and congratulate yourself on your achievement. You're learning how to delegate to your spouse or partner, allowing extra "me" time to exercise or just chill out. You're making better choices as you shop for food, as well as taking food to work and in the car as you run after active kids.

• If you don't have a family, then you and the 20-somethings have lots in common. You're seeking balance in a work-addicted world, and striving to remember to honor yourself as much as the people in your life that you care for. This week, recommit yourself to finding even more self-care time, and indulge in some new form of chilling out: that book you want to read, the DVD you're dying to see, or a museum you've been intending to visit. Nurture your mind as well as your body.

Mouth

• Feeding a family with so many different needs is like being a short-order cook. The key is to keep it simple. How many things can most of you share? Everyone needs steamed/roasted/grilled vegetables, so get them on the table. For the kids, cook vegetables into bread—zucchini bread, carrot muffins, whatever. Don't tell them it's healthy, just fun and delicious. Make fresh fruit smoothies instead of heavy calorie-laden desserts. See? It's food everyone can love.

Muscle

• If you've been compliant, by now you'll feel more energy and have greater endurance and strength. Look in the mirror. See any changes? Take out the tape measure and write down any reduction in inches. Sticking to your physical fitness guarantees you a smaller size at a higher-than-expected weight. Muscle weighs more than fat and takes up less space. Voilà—your hard work has paid off. With that renewed motivation, kick up your intensity and frequency even more. Come on, add some Vitamin-I and reenergize.

40s

Mind

• Your buffer zone for fooling around with your self-care and getting away with it has all but disappeared. This is not the time when you want to gain weight, since it's so much more difficult to remove it. That in and of itself is a great incentive not to stray too far from the path of wellness.

- Realize that six weeks of commitment are paying off. One of the greatest payoffs comes when your friends and colleagues note that somehow you're reversing the hands of time. Yes, it's true. You're looking younger. There's no more effective way to appear youthful and sustain it than to stick with a healthy lifestyle. You'll look like the mentally and physically fit man or woman you truly are.

Mouth

- Before you go out to dinner, have a mini-snack. If you're going to an evening eating event, curb your appetite by simply having a little something with protein in it. Eat one or two low-fat string cheese sticks or have a whole-wheat cracker spread with reduced-fat peanut butter. A small container of fat-free or low-fat yogurt or cottage cheese will also do it. This is especially true if the event is late in the evening. Remember, the later you eat, the lighter you eat!

Muscle

- How about using your newly emerging fitness for a good cause? There are countless 5K and 10K walks, runs, and bike rides that benefit charities. Choose one that's meaningful to you, and start to train for it now. What a gift for others—all because you decided to give to yourself. Fitness is the gift that keeps on giving.

50s

Mind

- After six weeks of being consistent, aiming for that 80 percent compliance I always espouse, you're noticing that chronic conditions like arthritis and lumbar pain are improving. You may also note that your mood is elevated and you've stopped withdrawing from social functions. Heck, you're starting to throw your own!

Mouth

- Try this experiment: One night, either by yourself or with your partner or friends, prepare dinner, put soothing background music on, dim the lights or light candles, and savor your dinner at a beautifully laid-out table—with absolutely no talking. That's right. It's a meditation dinner. You'll notice that without distractions and with full concentration on your meal, you'll eat less and enjoy it more. It's an amazing experience.

Muscle

- Test your newfound strength and endurance by seeing whether you can keep up with your grandchildren. Or, how about throwing the ball to your dog for an hour? Don't have the grocery-store boy help you with your bags; *you* lift them to your car. Need to haul compost for the garden? Not a problem. By the sixth week, you're one strong National Body Challenger!

60s and Beyond

Mind

- Since when is being 60 or 70 "old"? Not in your book! It's a state of mind and body. Science has clearly shown that as long as you routinely mind your self-care and combine it with lots of happy times, joy, and a saucy wit, you'll feel and look as youthful as you can be.

Mouth

- Taste and appetite can change as the digestive system goes through age-related transitions. You may find that some foods you used to enjoy are no longer as appetizing. This is your chance to try out new seasonings, spices, and sauces to enhance your meals.

Muscle

- National Institute of Aging researchers have found that around the seventh decade of life, the body begins to lose some muscle mass. That's why it's so very important to take your strength training seriously. This way, even when you lose some muscle mass, you haven't lost any significant strength. Utilize your weight training to stay strong and independent for years to come.

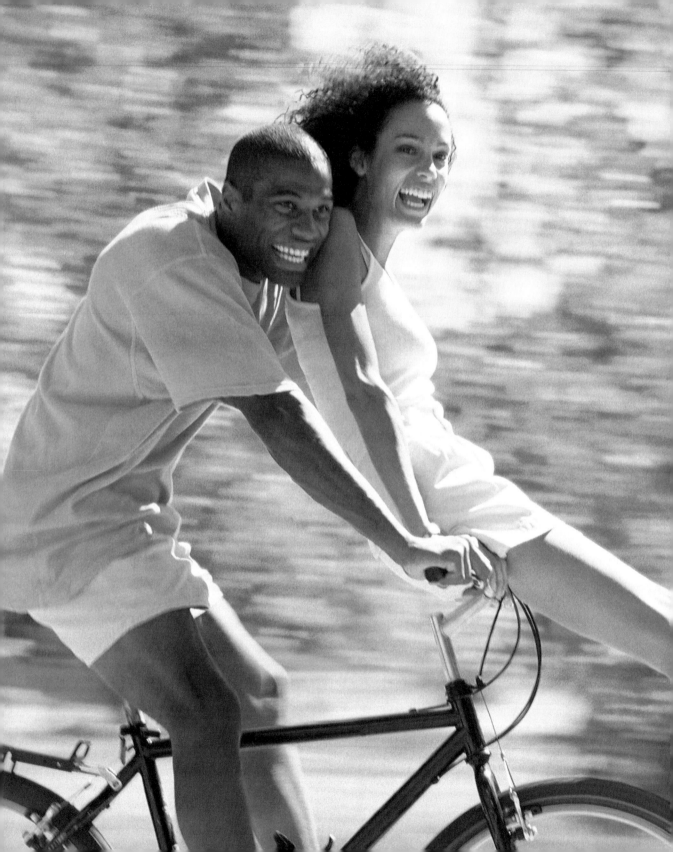

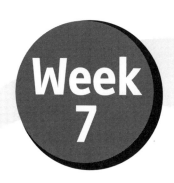

Week 7

Busting
Boredom

If you're doing the 8-week National Body Challenge, you have 2 weeks left. Regroup, and look at your progress so far. Hey, in 6 weeks you can really make a difference, can't you? If you followed my 80 percent rule and stuck to your Target Motivation, you should be proud of the changes you've made. So let's kick it up a notch and see what you can accomplish as you finish up these last 2 weeks.

If you were planning on doing the 12-week Challenge all along, then just continue to hammer away at your program, as you have another 6 weeks to go. Both groups can benefit from ramping up mindfulness, and practicing persistence and consistency in your newfound healthy lifestyle habits.

This week I want to bust through the boredom that can often happen after many weeks of hard work and effort. Someone in the family is definitely going to be feeling this way, and you all need to know how to help them. This happens faster with kids, most of whom have the attention span of a fly. So here are some tools to help all of you navigate through the boredom.

Week 7 Rules and Tools

Mind

- Boredom is actually a form of stress, caused by feeling as if you're not stimulated or contributing to the world in some meaningful way. Make a list of activities that have worked for you before, or those you really want to do but haven't yet. It could be anything from joining a hiking club to taking a college course. Choose one and make it happen this week.

- Get involved. Many communities offer opportunities for you to help with beautifying the landscape, maintaining walking trails, escorting kids on active outings, coaching a team, and so forth. The whole family can join in, and you'll be employing your new physical fitness for the good. That, in turn, will make you feel great. And I guarantee that you won't be bored!

Mouth

- Experiment with flavor. Try ethnic foods and new seasonings and condiments. Go vegetarian for a week. Every time you go to the market, buy one new fruit or vegetable that you've never eaten. Try a hybrid way of eating—become a "fish-vegetarian." It's easier to stay on track when you make eating more interesting.

- Take cooking classes; and learn how to make fun, exciting foods. Seek out a friend who's a fantastic cook and arrange to apprentice by her side, assisting and learning how to make that spectacular soup or fish fillet.

- Shake up where, how, and with whom you eat. New dishware, candles, or a floral arrangement on the table can spark up meals. How about inviting different folks into your life when you eat lunch at work or dinner at home? Spice up your conversations with a diversity of meal-time companions. In essence, turn eating into what it once was: engaging, personal, and nurturing, as well as delicious and satisfying.

Muscle

- Plan an active vacation. Choose a destination where you know there will be opportunities to move. Why not include a physical adventure such as hiking, biking, kayaking, horseback riding, mountain climbing, or skiing? Don't just sit under an umbrella watching the world go by.

- Explore new cardio options. You don't have to walk or run. Try out a rowing machine, an elliptical trainer, a stationary bike, or a stair climber. Cross-train by doing several different types of cardio workouts every week. Even trying different class instructors at your gym can jazz up your routine.

- Take the heart-rate challenge. Subtract your age from 220 and then aim for a heart rate that's 60 percent of that number for a moderate workout. Keep that heart rate for 10 to 15 minutes of your 30-minute workout. To add intensity, increase your heart rate to 70 percent. Once you do this for six to eight weeks, you can increase to 80 percent for five-minute intervals throughout your workout to achieve higher levels of aerobic fitness.

- Get into sports—and I don't mean watching them on TV! Tap in to your inner competitor by playing pick-up basketball or touch football in the park; or if you're into swimming, water polo. See if your work colleagues want to start a company softball team. Learn to play golf, racquetball, or badminton.

- Explore fun ways to move. When was the last time you played tether ball, dodge ball, or hacky sack with the kids or tossed a Frisbee for the dog? All types of physical activity result in more calories burned and can make life more enjoyable.

- Even when the weather's bad, you can still be active indoors. Play table tennis, pool, foosball, or darts. Go dancing: try swing, salsa, ballroom, or hip-hop. Anything that keeps you up and moving is better than slumping in front of the TV or computer screen.

It's a Generational Thing

Kids 7–12

Mind

- It's all about color. Make a list of six colorful vegetables you'll eat this week. Have one or both of your parents sit at the computer with you as you log on to **www.discoveryhealth.com** and click onto the Nutrition and Fitness Center to learn what kinds of vitamins and nutrients are in each one, and what they can do for you.

Mouth

- Your challenge this week is to make sure to have three colors of vegetables in your sandwich, salad, and on your dinner plate. Tell Mom and Dad that you need to be doing this whenever you eat throughout the day.

Muscle

- Make a list of activities you like to do—walking, running, playing basketball, or roller skating, for example. Log on to **http://discovery health.com/tools/calculators/activity/activity.html** to get some other ideas and learn how many calories you're burning when you do these activities for one hour. It's your goal to do one hour of physical activity every day. With your help, we'll just make sure to keep it interesting!

Mind

• If you've been hitting your target most of the time, the changes you're seeing are usually incentive enough to continue going. If even small changes stuck, you can still see enough of a difference in six weeks to make you smile. So fuel up on feeling good about your accomplishments so far and keep on keepin' on.

• If you started this with a poor sense of self-esteem, take a moment and assess how you feel now. Doing better? You're experiencing a mental and physical transformation that's going to help get you through the emotional and hormonal roller coaster of adolescence. This transformation goes on for a lifetime, and allows you to keep growing mentally, physically, and spiritually.

Mouth

• Yes, it's still hard to avoid the junk food that seems to be everywhere all the time. And maybe by now you're feeling a bit bored eating the same old healthy choices. Break out of your food rut by experimenting with healthy foods you normally don't eat. Include soy products in your proteins this week, including energy bars and shakes. How about flavored, low-calorie sports drinks if you find it hard to get your water in each day? Find one new restaurant that serves a healthy menu alternative. Make that your weekly homework.

Muscle

• Continuing interest springs from challenge. Try new sports and movement techniques. If you're 18 and over, ask your parents if you can join a health club with lots of different offerings. If you're under 18 and your parents' health club has a family day, go along and take advantage of it. You're lookin' good. Let's keep it up!

20s

Mind

- Find a day spa where you can experience total relaxation through a body wrap, aromatherapy massage, or healing facial. It's important to honor opportunities to get that mental rest to keep your Target Motivation focus fresh in your mind as you continue your healthy lifestyle habits.

Mouth

- Going to the same boring restaurants? How about learning how to cook tasty, healthy fare at home. Invite a slew of friends over to enjoy it with you. For that matter, have them cook one side dish each and add this to your main entree. Now you've instigated a fantastic party . . . and perhaps a regular ritual!

Muscle

- Instead of pounding out time on your treadmill or cross trainer with the same old music, download some hot new tunes into your MP3 player, and step it up!

30s

Mind

- During these past six weeks, you've discovered your strengths and vulnerabilities when it comes to sticking to a healthy lifestyle. Look at the three elements Mind, Mouth, and Muscle. See if that Target Motivation is keeping you going through your hectic days. Refresh it if you need to. Let's look at the other two elements and continue to refine to keep the momentum going.

Mouth

- To create a balance in your dietary intake, it's important to incorporate healthy pleasures. There's nothing wrong with an occasional glass of wine with dinner, a cookie with tea in the afternoon, or a lunch with friends. Just not every day and as long as you're working it off with physical activity at some point.

160   **The National Body Challenge Success Program for the Whole Family**

- For you 30-something women, when PMS hits, how about creating a PMS jar? Put a 2-oz serving of your favorite PMS food (licorice twists, cookies, candy) into it to use it when you need to get it out of your system. (If necessary, put it in a Ziploc baggie to keep it fresh.) It has to be a nonbingeable food.

- For you pregnant ladies or new moms, be mindful of eating fresh, whole foods in *woman-size* portions as you transition from pregnant to postpartum and beyond. This is especially important if you're breast-feeding and you want your milk to provide high-quality meals for your baby.

Muscle

- How does your exercise regimen feel to you right now? Is it beginning to feel like it's a piece of you? I'll bet you know by now how much that walk or workout helps you maintain your sanity when you're feeling so overwhelmed by life.

- Are your kids complaining that "there's nothing to do"? Come up with some active games you can play to break up family boredom, like treasure or scavenger hunts. Introduce the kids to some old-fashioned activities like sack or three-legged races.

40s

Mind

- Look over your journals. How is your motivation? Has it changed at all? What have your learning experiences, mistakes, and triumphs taught you about attaining and maintaining a healthy lifestyle? Make a list of at least three items you've incorporated into your life in the Mind, Mouth, and Muscle categories. If you're doing the eight-week Challenge, then continue to refine your initial three, and plan on adding to this list for months to come as you continue this lifelong journey. Twelve-weekers, your challenge is to achieve three more over the next six weeks.

Mouth

- Hippocrates said, "Let food be thy medicine." Well, it's time to understand what he was talking about. Log on to **www.discoveryhealth. com**, click on "Nutrition Index," and learn why healthy foods work for you as you strive to prevent or treat medical conditions. You'll see that your foods should indeed be your medicine cabinet of wondrous anti-oxidants and healing nutrients.

Muscle

- To safely increase your intensity this week, try a "walk and jog." As long as your weight-bearing joints are in good shape, walk for five minutes and jog for one to two minutes. If that feels comfortable, then start alternating walking and jogging. This will save your knees from the constant battering of running.

- Men tend to get right into weight training. Women often defer to cardio as strength training is foreign territory, especially for you 40-somethings. Well, get over it: It's imperative that you strength-train as you cross into your 40s. You should have started it by at least the second or third week. If not, start now.

- Women, you may need someone to show you the right form, which will help you maximize weight loss and avoid injury. Consider taking a class at the YWCA, watch a video, or work with a trainer at the gym. Lift weights twice a week, and remember to be patient. You don't build muscles overnight.

50s

Mind

- Take heart in the fact that even you 50-year-olds can see striking changes in your bodies if you simply stay consistent. Your patience pays off as you see inches coming off, body fat burned, and greater physical independence and function. Well done! Make sure to keep your expectations of this mental and physical transformation realistic. There's no overnight or radical change going on here, nor should there ever be . . . just patient nurturing and refining.

Mouth

- This week, be a teacher. Offer your kids and friends healthy eating advice as well as recipes you've learned over the past six weeks. Cook together and talk about the experience. Make "see one, do one, teach one" your mantra. By doing so, it keeps you fresh and up-to-date about healthy cooking.

Muscle

• Once, the 50s were when you were supposed to settle back, relax, and watch the world go by. No more! They're all about renewal as you go forth and use that fit body to explore the world. Remember, Helen Keller said, "Life is either a daring adventure or nothing at all." This is a key "daring-adventure" time of life. Surfing, sky diving, parasailing, and kayaking await!

60s and Beyond

Mind

• You might hear others noting that once you're 60 there's no point in pushing your envelope. Well, you've just proved them wrong. Now you know that age has nothing to do with the ability to achieve and sustain a healthier body, no matter when you started the journey. You can be fitter, stronger, sexier, and happier than you've ever been, if you believe you can. First believe, then achieve, and finally succeed.

Mouth

• Want a simple, healthy, and tasty way to prepare lunch or dinner? Learn how to make soup and combine it with a delicious salad. Remember, 60-year-olds don't need a mountain of food. Log on to **http://discoveryhealth.foodfit.com** and you'll find great recipes for preparing these simple yet life-giving dishes.

Muscle

• I challenge you to look online for a fantastic, doable, and safe way to celebrate your newfound fitness. How about signing up for a Country Walkers vacation either in the U.S. or abroad? You'll be surrounded by like-minded individuals full of energy and a zest for living well. If you've been doing your 10,000 steps daily and continuing your strength, flexibility, and balance exercises, then you're set to go.

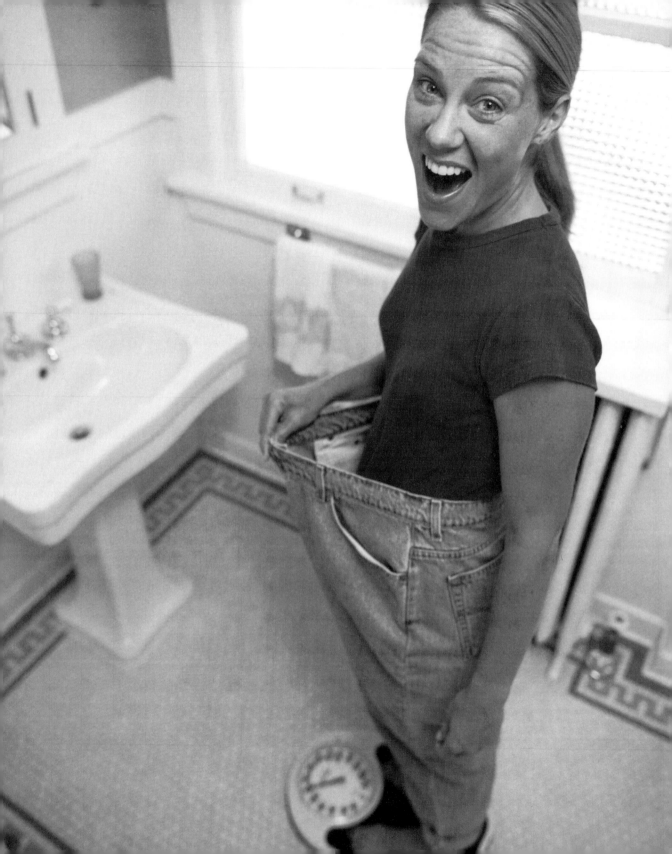

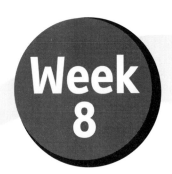

A
Taste *of*
Triumph

For all of you, whether you're 8- or 12-week National Body Challengers, it's an amazing accomplishment to complete 8 weeks, or 2 months, of hard work. If you wondered how much anyone could achieve in this time period, then just whip out your tape measure, get your body fat rechecked, slip on your "clothes-o-meter," and see how you've done compared to how you were at the beginning. Celebrate all changes, whether large or small.

Look back and reread your first words as you embraced this Challenge. Take a moment to reflect on, and appreciate, your efforts. Realize how a correct mind-set, the right Target Motivation, and a belief in yourself all helped you achieve a powerful and sustainable mental and physical transformation.

Take your old, larger clothes that no longer fit and give them to a charity that will recycle them for the needy. When you give them away, know that you're not going back to that size again. Have a little celebration by getting new clothes that reflect your healthy outlook and way of living.

If you've reached a body-fat percentage and size that works for you, from now on the clothes you wear every day *are* your "clothes-o-meter." Once you've achieved your optimal body composition, you know that if your clothing becomes too tight, you need to rein in your eating and bump up your physical activity.

For once, celebrate without raiding the fridge. Head off to the department store and ask a personal shopper or clerk to help you with a new look. Guys, get rid of the baggy pants and buy a new belt. Ladies, run from elastic and start to seek out tailored looks that keep you on the straight and—literally!—narrow! Kids, it's time to hop into those cool clothes you wanted to wear to school. You all deserve a round of applause!

If you had medical conditions and were on medications at the start, reassess each with your physician. One of the greatest rewards for consistent self-care is your ability to reduce or eliminate medications, and moreover, either prevent or reverse a medical condition such as heart disease, high blood pressure, or diabetes.

You will take this achievement and keep practicing what you've learned for the rest of your life. Recall that the purpose of this Challenge was to teach you how to live well. You have tools that will always be available to you as you learn more, refine your habits, and keep pace with your own unique aging process. We will always be here to partner with you, providing you with cutting-edge science and then showing you simple applications for your daily lives. Just log on to **www.discoveryhealth.com** and click on to the National Body Challenge for the Rules and Tools of this lifelong wellness journey.

Week 8 Rules and Tools

Mind

- Get a positive "bodytude"! That means embracing your accomplishments and not diminishing them based upon unrealistic expectations. Substitute "but" with "and." At the end of a Challenge, it's common for people to say, "I removed 15 pounds, *but* I should have removed more." No, celebrate your wonderful achievement and instead say: "I removed 15 pounds, *and* I'm going to continue this journey until I reach my goal." Now, you're talkin'! Go around to each family member who participated, and make sure they all get this message. Celebrate as a family.

• Recognize the power of the mind-body connection. What secured your success in the Challenge was the right mind-set, which then made it easier to start the technical work of executing the healthy eating and physical activity. Look at that Target Motivation right now. You may have already achieved enough to make it necessary to develop a new one for yourself. Realize that this Challenge was a holistic, integrative program, driven by the Mind, and interacting with Mouth and Muscle. This is your blueprint for healthy living. You get to have the fun and enjoyment of customizing it to your unique lifestyle needs.

• Reward yourself for your achievement with a body gift. How about a soothing sports or aromatherapy massage, or an energizing Thai massage and bodywork. Bask in the wonderful relaxation of this reward.

Mouth
• Marvel about how your tastes, portion sizes, and the quality of your food have changed in these eight weeks. There *is* life after minimizing or eliminating all of the processed and refined foods you used to swear you couldn't live without. In eight weeks, you taught your body to crave healthier alternatives. Well done!

• Make a list of what you'd like to refine now as you continue this Challenge. You see, it's always something. You'll constantly tweak your eating habits, always looking for newer, healthy foods as you shop. You'll find that there are challenging times in your life when eating well seems like a mission impossible. Deadlines, family crises, and job stresses are all major speed bumps on the road to wellness. Take a deep breath and learn how to navigate them without spending body dollars and resorting to self-destructive behaviors. Regroup and do the best you can. Men and women who do so . . . look and feel like it.

Muscle
• Record your new levels of physical endurance, strength, and flexibility. The body is so forgiving of the weeks, months, and years of neglect. In eight weeks your body adapted to your increased activity . . . and guess

what? There's more where that came from. Don't stop now. Keep pushing the envelope. Keep your physical activity dynamic. Constantly look for ways to challenge yourself. That sense of accomplishment will be a source of greater motivation to keep the challenge going—*for life.*

• Look at your body differently now. Perhaps you were using derogatory language when you referred to it. Your self-image was poor. You feared the loss of independence as you aged. Things are happily different now. By gradually increasing your physical fitness, you can now walk at a brisker pace, bike, and hike—without so many aches and pains. And you can keep up with the kids, climb those stairs more easily, and hoist that luggage into the rack on the plane. You're functioning at a higher level and enjoying life more.

• Doing your walks and staying strong and flexible are now integral parts of your life. Incorporate more of your new physical fitness into your day. Why not take those stairs at the office, or get up and walk around during work hours? How about forming an exercise group at work so you and your co-workers can help keep each other on track? After all, you're now an inspiration to others. Living an active lifestyle is the gift that keeps on giving, as you motivate others to do the same.

It's a Generational Thing

Kids 7–12

Mind

• So how does it feel? This is like finishing a tough class at school and getting through it. But hey, the learning doesn't just stop here. You're officially enrolled in the School of You. This is a lifelong course, and the good news is that it gets easier with practice. Look to your parents to help guide you through the coming weeks, months, and years. Heck, when they look like they're having a tough time, why don't you inspire *them?* You see, it will always be a family affair!

Mouth

- I'm giving you some fair warning here. It will continue to be a growing challenge to find ways to avoid the temptation to go back to unhealthy eating habits. You're surrounded with such temptations when you're visiting friends, going to the mall or movies, or when you're at school. Just remember that it's perfectly okay to have a treat every now and then. But you'll feel and look better if you work hard to choose healthier foods most of the time.

Muscle

- I'll bet you feel lighter and more energized now that you're more fit and have dropped some of that body fat. Keep looking for ways to stay active. Hang out with kids who like to get out and throw the ball, bike, roller blade, or run. Play sports or do martial arts. Trust me when I tell you that by doing this you will feel better about yourself, do better in school, enjoy improved relationships with friends and family, and look terrific. What a deal!

Teens 13–19

Mind

- So what did you accomplish over these eight weeks? Remember, don't minimize any achievement. You're probably feeling less down on yourself about your body. Terrific! And you realize that your physical fitness makes you proud of yourself. Well done! And you realize that guys like gals who are together in mind, body, and spirit, and the same is true for the way gals view guys.

  It's not just the appearance thing. That's empty and vacuous. The real winners are well-rounded teens whose source of pride in themselves stems from the meaningful things (good grades, sports, volunteering) they do in their lives, and not from obsessing about the scale or a dress size. Healthy teens are beautiful inside and out. You've achieved this goal during your National Body Challenge. Now run with this—*for life.*

Mouth

- You're curbing your intake of sugar and colas, rarely eating fried foods, prioritizing chicken and fish over burgers, and having one or two slices of pizza instead of the whole thing. I say you're well on the way to establishing healthy, realistic eating habits. Keep finding ways to chip away at these daily challenges.

Muscle

- As you transition through high school and on to college, make it a habit to walk everywhere you can, and sign up for activities that will keep you active and engaged. You'll perform better in school if you stay active. You already know this, since you've had eight weeks to experience this effect. It's a mind-body connection that will keep you calm and sane throughout life's endless struggles and triumphs.

20s

Mind

- I hope you see by now that despite living the single life, running around trying to find that perfect mate, getting through college and perhaps professional school, living away from home for the first time, and starting out in the workforce, you really can integrate some meaningful lifestyle changes and keep 'em up. Seeing is believing, and you've just experienced eight weeks of new, healthy living. Tremendous!

Mouth

- Dashboard dining, grab-and-go, and meal skipping were your standard operating procedures when you started the National Body Challenge. You may still grab and run out the door, but you're smarter about your choices now—for example, low-fat cheese, sprouts, and tomato in a pita with an apple instead of the scone or croissant. You see, it's all about customizing your habits to your 20-something active lifestyle. It's totally possible to live through your 20s and hold on to a healthy lifestyle. You're living proof!

Muscle

• By now you've made it clear to all of your friends and colleagues that you don't blow off your exercise routine. And, for that matter, you're asking them to join you so you can talk about work or personal issues. Racquetball and tennis courts, golf ranges, or the gym all become the new hangouts for 20-year-old men and women who are clued into wellness.

30s

Mind

• Give yourself a serious high five. Despite growing career pressures, and starting relationships and families, you persevered. What a tremendous accomplishment. This is the one decade when all heck is breaking out in your social, personal, and professional life. And you still managed to hang in there. Make a list of your accomplishments, and revel in the fact that you did this against the odds. Well done!

Mouth

• Feeding a family of any size, whether you're a couple or you've got three kids in tow, will continue to be a challenge as you try to keep your own healthy eating in focus. Remember the rule: The more complex your life is, the simpler you have to keep the eating. By now, you've spent eight weeks experimenting and developing the easiest way to feed your self when life is frantic. Spend another eight weeks refining this and showing how well you can demonstrate flexibility as your life continues to evolve.

Muscle

• Keep finding ways to share family activities. For eight weeks you've been learning how to be creative. Family hikes and outings are a great way to have fun and show the kids that a healthy, active lifestyle is the way to go. Meanwhile, you need to keep paying attention to your own personal regimen. Continue to get up early and get in that cardio workout. Make it to your strength-training sessions twice per week. You may have to wedge it in between family obligations, but that's a small price to pay to have so many wonderful people in your life!

40s

Mind

• What a gift you've given yourself by completing these eight weeks: the gift of longevity and wellness. You're at a stage when you finally have to take your health and well-being seriously—and you did! You rose to the occasion and slugged it out, facing off with the demons of your unhealthy habits, and slowly but surely substituting them with new, healthy ones. You're reading more about how lifestyle affects disease risk, and you know that at the end of the day, you're actively taking steps to save your own life. That has to make you feel pretty darned proud of yourself.

Mouth

• Whether you're a man or woman, the party is now officially over: You can't continue to overeat and get away with it. Before you joined the National Body Challenge, you were pushing the envelope, winging it on your eating and hoping you didn't gain much weight. Well, once you crossed 40, your random lifestyle habits were no longer working. You were gaining weight and feeling down about it. These eight weeks taught you that by paying more attention to the quality, quantity, and frequency of your eating, you were able to reverse the weight gain, get your girth under control, and feel energized.

Muscle

• Daily physical activity is now officially nonnegotiable. No more excuses or complaining. It's over. You've been incorporating this into your life no matter what. You realize that true balance in your life comes from a healthy, realistic attitude combined with good nutrition and an active lifestyle. After eight weeks, you're convinced that this great feeling from putting it all together is priceless—and that your very life depends on keeping it up.

50s

Mind

• Your old "I can't do this" attitude has now been replaced by an assertive "can do" mental state. This is the end of feeling hopeless, helpless, and defeated when applied to changing your mind and body. *Of course* you can move more and take charge of your nutrition. Your changes over these past eight weeks may have been significant enough to result in fewer medications, or the complete elimination of some or all of your drugs, as well as prevention or reversal of actual medical conditions. Celebrate every one of these victories. If you're almost there, keep chipping away. Repeat the Challenge as many times as it takes to achieve your goals.

Mouth

• Eating has now become a more sensual and pleasurable experience. You have the time and wherewithal to find and prepare the healthiest foods. You've made the healthy food/healthy life connection, and you're practicing this every day. You're finally honoring your body, and nourishing it with foods that fuel and bring pleasure and joy to your palate.

Muscle

• By now you've completely dismissed the idea that age limits your ability to reverse a previously sedentary lifestyle. For that matter, you're continuing to try out new ways to push your physical limits. You're discovering the utter pleasure of doing things you thought you could never do—such as running that 5K or hiking up Kilimanjaro. And you know that for every step you take and every weight you lift, you're that much further from disease risk, and that much closer to a longer life of wellness.

60s and Beyond

Mind

• You thought that the National Body Challenge was for the younger folks. And you proved yourself wrong. I hope you're absolutely amazed by how your body can reverse a history of sedentary habits and overeating. Moreover, do you see the effect on your mind? You men and women 60 and beyond are living proof that learning to live a healthier lifestyle isn't restricted to any age group. It's an ageless process. The mind and body are wonderfully forgiving and just waiting for you to take charge and make changes. Congratulations on your success thus far, and here's to repeating your Challenge again and again as you refine your lifestyle skills and find new ways to feel joy in your daily living.

Mouth

- After eight weeks, you've seen how eating whole foods appropriately can help reverse medical conditions (diabetes, high cholesterol) while improving energy levels and overall functioning. Preparing healthy foods is a loving ritual for yourself and your loved ones. Junk food, overeating, and skipping meals have no place in the life of a man or woman who embraces life the way that you do now.

Muscle

- The National Body Challenge has convinced you that youthfulness is a state of mind. You're more physically independent, functioning at higher levels, and reveling in your new strength and endurance. In only eight weeks, you can see amazing changes in your ability to get around and caregive others. Your regular regimen of cardio and weight training is protecting you from ending up in a hospital with a broken hip because you weren't strong enough to handle a fall. Your body is fitter, which has made your mind sharper and your memory crisper.

  At the end of the day, you finally realize that the National Body Challenge has taught you that the best caregiver is a healthy caregiver—to you, to your spouse, kids, and those grandkids who want you around forever. Well, maybe not forever, but for a very long and joyful time!

Onward and Upward

Those of you who feel like you want to continue the National Body Challenge, go right ahead. Repeat the last four weeks and make it a full 12-week Challenge if you want. In one more month you might be able to fully achieve your goals. Here are some rules and tools for adding the extra four weeks to your National Body Challenge:

If you've reached a plateau, then first add Vitamin-I to your exercise. Increase the intensity of your workouts, concentrating on form, and adding as much challenge (hills, speed, weight) as you can tolerate. Then be careful about how much you're eating. Often you're unaware that you're eating more than you need. Count calories, and see where you can tighten up your dietary intake.

When stress gets to you and threatens to derail your efforts, practice regrouping. Transition from Plan A to Plan B, C, or Z if you need to. Your life will present endless chances to regroup. Expect tough times, and embrace them as opportunities to practice stress-resilient regrouping.

Keep your eye on the goal. Sharpen your Target Motivation so that it's an effective guide during difficult times.

Get that support system in place to help you finish your Challenge and achieve your goals. Family members, colleagues, and friends are all great sources of loving cheerleading to spur you along to success.

I encourage you to revisit this program as many times as you need to in order to achieve your goals. That is, repeat the Challenge as many times as you want. Life presents situations where weight gain is inevitable—perhaps physical disability or taking medications. Just come back to the National Body Challenge and reconnect to get back to your healthy body composition.

Now you have the basics to keep you and your family on the path to love, joy, and wellness!

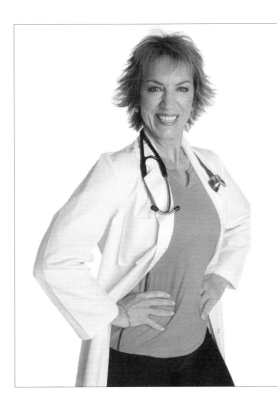

PART III

Success Stories of Physical and Mental Transformations

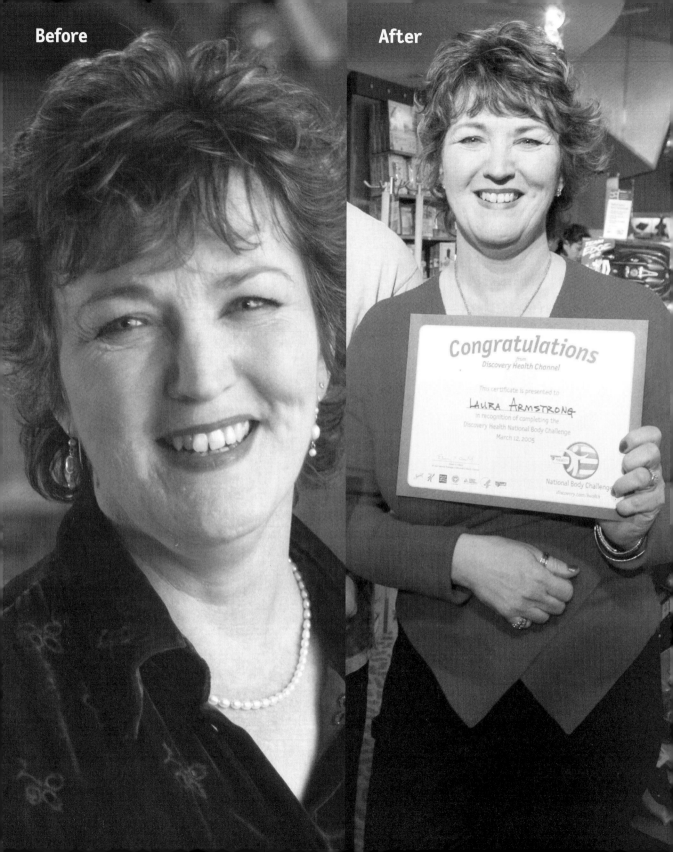

Before

After

Laura Armstrong Is a Goal-Getter

Like a lot of you, Laura Armstrong, a 48-year-old mother of two boys and a senior manager at a trade association, had packed on weight after her pregnancies. "Probably about 20 pounds per baby," she says. When she started the Challenge she was peaking at 182 pounds. "My normal fighting weight before I was married was about 140. I had just gotten a lot fatter than I realized."

Laura read about the National Body Challenge online and decided to go for it. Her husband accompanied her to Pentagon City Mall near her Arlington, Virginia, home to register at the Discovery Channel Store there. "My husband is a basketball nut; he plays three or four times a week," she remarks. "He's always been very athletic and fortunately, both my children take after him in terms of build. So it was hard for him to watch me get to the state I was in." He could have given her advice, she admits, "but if he wanted to stay married, he knew he couldn't tell me what to do!"

Still, it was her husband who prodded Laura into taking the National Body Challenge. When she saw the crowds at the store, she had some misgivings about identifying herself with them. "Even though they were people like me with the same goals, it was a little bit intimidating to realize that I'd gotten to that stage, that I was one of them." She also didn't want all those people knowing how much she weighed. "So I said to my husband, 'I don't think I'm going to do this,' and he said, 'Yes, you are.' And there we are hissing back and forth at each other. Finally, he made me mad enough that I said, 'Oh, all right.'"

After Laura was recruited to participate in the 2004 televised Challenge, her family became her cheerleaders. "Throughout the whole process, I had the support of my guys like you wouldn't believe," she says. "All three of them were very, very enthusiastic."

I worked with Laura as well as Brian Ross and Beth Powell, all of whom shared their daily lifestyle changes both on Discovery Health Channel's Website as well as the television show.

Mind

Laura cites her weight as her primary motivation for taking the Challenge. "I didn't like the way I looked; I didn't like the way I felt," she says. But there was an even more important consideration that she'd been avoiding dealing with. She had high blood pressure. Her mother died of heart disease, and within the last three years her father had a quintuple bypass.

"So I've got a genetic double-whammy on that," she says. "It was an issue I'd skated around for a long time, but with the onset of age—oh my gosh, I'm going to be 50 in a couple of years!—I thought I might as well face it now."

Mouth

"I'm a chocoholic; I could be counted on to put away a box of Oreos," says Laura. We explained to her that smart eating isn't about deprivation. She could have a piece of chocolate when she really wanted one as long as she worked it into her overall plan and it didn't lead to bingeing. Eat it, enjoy it, and then get back on the program. "I think that if they hadn't given me permission to eat the chocolate, I would have gone ahead and done it anyway but felt bad," she says. "But then I found that the less I ate of the really sugary stuff, the less I wanted it. I'd always heard that, but didn't really believe it was true."

Laura also benefited from completing the food logs we had her hand in every week. "In the beginning, I had no idea how much I was eating, and I thought I was doing pretty well until I started adding it up," she says. "So the food log was very important."

Once she started eating five or six small, balanced meals a day, she says, "I needed it less because I got to where I could do it without thinking about it." Based upon her Resting Metabolic Rate, she stuck to 1,400 to 1,600 calories per day and aimed to burn 300 to 400 calories during daily physical activity.

Now it's become second nature. Just recently she went on a two-week annual event that her company puts on out of town. "The dinners every night are huge and lengthy, with lots of alcohol" she says. "There's just so much, but I actually lost a couple of pounds there this time. I knew what to eat, and I knew when to stop eating."

Muscle

Laura uses the gym in her condo building now, even though she hadn't taken advantage of the facilities in the entire ten years she lived there up till now. It sure was handy when we started her on her daily cardio regimen. "I would get up early, take myself downstairs, slap on the headphones, and just go for it," she says. She primarily used the treadmill, but would occasionally take on the elliptical trainer, even though she didn't like it as much, because she knew mixing it up would keep her metabolism humming. Since then, she's joined a gym in her office building—which she'd also never used before—and discovered the rowing machine. "I love it," she says. "I come off there feeling like I've really done a lot of work in a short amount of time." That's Vitamin I = Intensity at work.

Laura found that regular exercise had a big impact on her life. "In my office, they could see better than I could the effect it was having on me. With all the exercise, I was a lot less stressed, which of course, makes you better to be around."

Her Proudest Achievement

"You mean apart from my being able to see my waist again and my pants falling off my hips?" Laura asks, laughing.

That actually would be enough for some people, but for Laura it was "a shift in perception that I was someone who could do this. We all complain that we need to take off weight, and suddenly I was someone who actually was, and who was sticking with it, and who was becoming a role model." She's particularly proud about being an example for her sons. "My guys seeing me doing this and know now that it doesn't matter how old you are—and they think I'm older than dirt! If you make up your mind to do something, you stick with it, you use the resources you have available, and then you can do anything."

There's something else. Her blood pressure is down. "My doctor said, 'It's very rare for me to see people come in healthier than they were the year before,'" says Laura. "That really made me feel proud, too."

Her Best Tip

Buddy up. Try to take the Challenge with somebody who isn't going to nag you, who has the same goals, and needs the same support that you do. "It's not just about them providing support to you," says Laura, "but you providing support to them, too. The more you have invested in other people, the more you have invested in yourself."

Laura considers herself lucky to have gone through the Challenge with Brian and Beth. "We still think of ourselves as a team," she says. "While we don't work out together, we do e-mail and call each other, and I think that's as important as physically being in the same room and sweating together."

Height: 5'7"	8-Week Program	
	Before	**After**
Weight:	177	158
Waist size:	37"	33.4"
BMI:	27.7	25
Body fat:	37.5%	31.5%
Total Pounds Removed:	19	

Her Future Plans

Laura's goal is to continue removing weight until she reaches 145 to 150 pounds. "I was comfortable and looked pretty darn good at that weight, if I say so myself!" she says. In addition, she wants to see if keeping the weight off will also keep her blood pressure down to the point that she no long requires medication. "That can only be a good thing, for me and for my family," she says.

Remember how I told you that the physical changes you experience will lead to other profound changes? This is what Laura discovered, too. "There are things I want to do in life, and in some twisted way I was using 40 extra pounds as an excuse not to do them, and an excuse to believe that I couldn't," she says. "I had let myself go in more ways than physically. Seeing that I can remove the weight has given me the courage to consider that I can achieve those other goals as well, if that's what I want to do.

"This all has a trickle-down effect. If my kids and others see that I can achieve these goals, knowing me as they do, it might sink in that they can achieve their dreams as well."

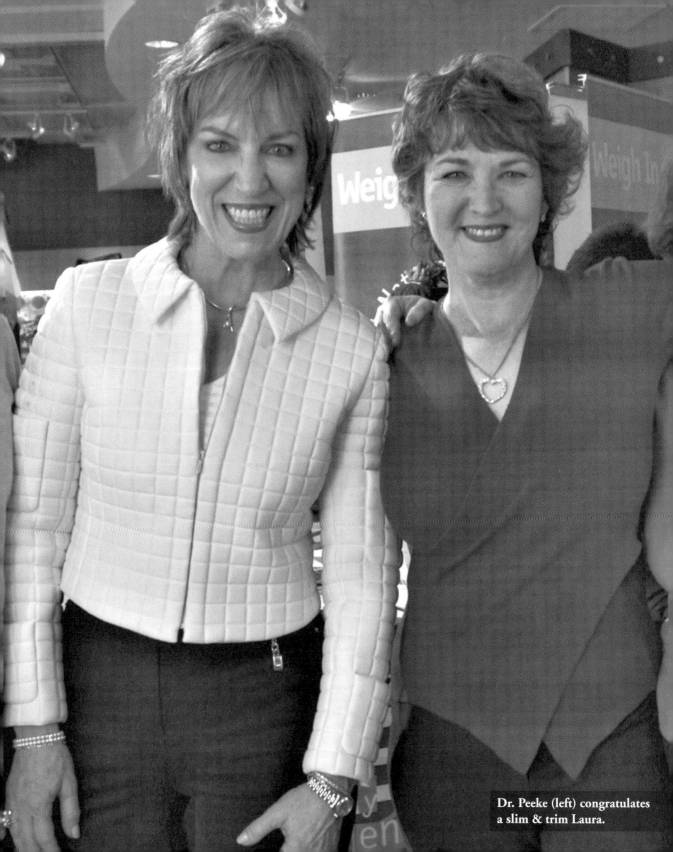

Dr. Peeke (left) congratulates
a slim & trim Laura.

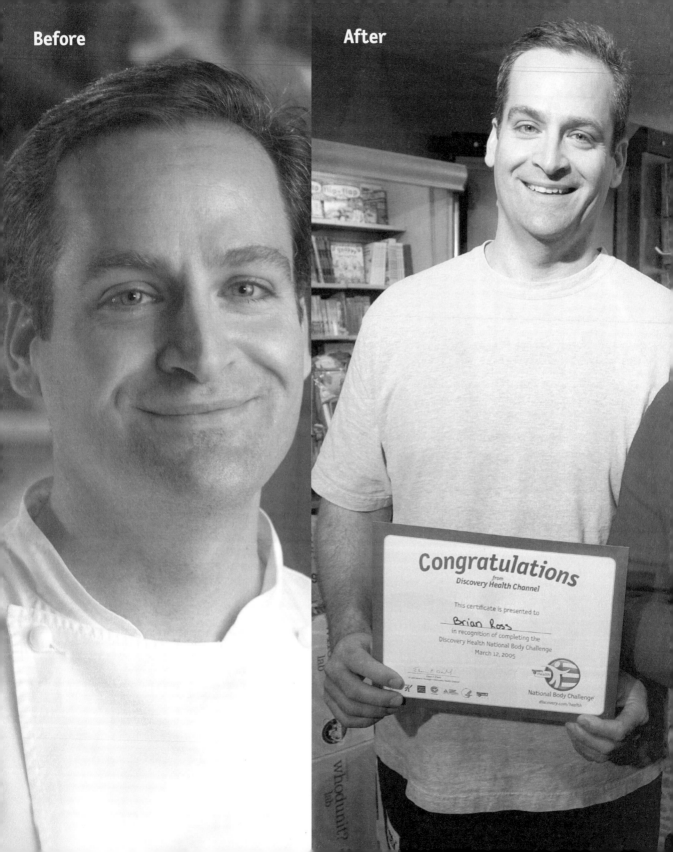

Before

After

Brian Ross
Cooks!

Talk about challenges. Chef Brian Ross, 41, had plenty when he started his program in January 2005. He teaches at a culinary school in Bethesda, Maryland. "On any given day, I've got anywhere from 15 to 30 students cooking food that I taste," he says. Also, he says, "We've got a full-time pastry program and have Danish and cookies and cakes lying around." And there were even more cookies on the menu at home, where he had a toddler and a pregnant wife.

Understandably, battling weight wasn't a new thing for Brian. "For me, historically, I've sometimes eaten well, but the exercise portion wasn't where it should be, and I had moderately successful results," he says. "Then there were other times when I ate whatever I wanted, but I was active on the treadmill, and I maintained but didn't do any better. This National Body Challenge was the first time that everything was happening at once." He's talking, of course, about the Mind, Mouth, and Muscle formula.

Mind

The first few weeks on the program, this man who had never been particularly active and had "always been chubby," battled through record-breaking snowstorms to get to the gym. "It was hard sometimes with the young baby and my wife getting morning sickness, but she was very supportive because we knew it was important," he says.

Why so important? Brian was finally motivated to make changes for health reasons. "I didn't have full-blown anything," he says. But his weight had reached a lifetime peak. "My blood pressure was elevated, and my cholesterol was the highest it had ever been," he says. "My knees were really starting to hurt me, and I was getting fed up with being tired all the time."

When he began, his body fat was 33.8 percent; his BMI, 32.4; and his muscle mass, 158 pounds. All had room for improvement. Before the Challenge, Brian's cholesterol was 185; after, it was 153. As Brian sustains his healthy lifestyle, he could keep himself off medication in the future. A recent study from the School of Dietetics and Human Nutrition at McGill University in Canada showed that a healthy diet can lower total cholesterol and LDL ("bad" cholesterol), and exercise can increase HDL ("good" cholesterol) and lower triglyceride levels to the point that they can replace medications for people with slightly elevated cholesterol levels. We also measured his body composition using a high-tech body comp analyzer. His blood pressure was down, too. "My knees didn't hurt anymore, my clothes fit, I was standing up straighter, and I felt terrific."

And that's what it's all about.

Mouth

Brian had already determined to shed some weight even before he joined the National Body Challenge. He'd removed 13 pounds by cutting back on calories, but was doing no exercise. He decided to join the National Body Challenge to take advantage of the trial gym membership, but he got a lot more!

Like the other Challengers, Brian underwent high tech: We first measured his resting metabolic rate, which tells us how many calories he needed just to stay at his current weight. Then we figured that he should be eating approximately 2,100 to 2,300 calories per day to begin to remove excess body fat. But we tried to keep his six meals at around 2,000, giving him 100 to 300 extra for that tasting in the classroom. (Now that's a great example of how the program can be personalized to fit your lifestyle.) He also used his cooking expertise to come up with healthy recipes that he shared on the show.

Muscle

"I was not in very good shape," admits Brian. "Truthfully, I had not been very active." Before he met with trainer Jason Hadeed, who started him on strength training and supervised his cardio workouts, we directed Brian to just get cracking on one hour of cardio every day. The key was Vitamin I = Intensity. The more intense his workout, the more calories he would burn and the more body fat he'd remove.

"I did the elliptical trainer because that was a little bit easier on my knees," he says. This was the start of a lifestyle change: In eight weeks he missed only two days of cardio. Once he added two weight-training sessions a week and then doubled that at Week 4, the effort began to show results. At three weeks he'd removed about 6 pounds, at six weeks it was at 16, and by the end he was down 19 pounds. "But that was just scale weight," Brian stresses. As well as removing fat, he gained fat-free mass (muscle).

His Proudest Achievement

Passing it forward was Brian's proudest achievement. He and his wife now both have gym memberships, a great example for their growing family. He has also started teaching a healthy cooking class. "I was standing up there in front of 30 paying customers, preaching the gospel of 'Take care of your body,'" he says. "They were asking me questions, and I was saying, 'Well, this is what *I* do.'" Brian is now the chef who walks the talk.

His Best Tip

Don't reward success with failure. The most dangerous point, he says, is around Week 6 when you can see results. "Your pants fit, and people start telling you how good you look." That's when it's tempting to say, "I'll be fine; I don't need to stay the course all the time now. The bottom line is that this can't be a temporary thing." Indeed, this is a lifelong journey.

His Future Plans

Brian's goals are to keep on removing excess fat until he reaches a body-fat percentage somewhere between 20 and 25. He wants his waist size to be closer to 36" and definitely no more than 38". That's because he knows that in men, a girth of 40" or more is associated with an increased risk of diabetes, heart disease, and colon cancer. Finally, he wants to keep practicing his healthy lifestyle with his family in order to integrate this lifestyle, and to teach his children that it's possible to live well and sustain it—*for life*.

Height: 6'	8-Week Program	
	Before	After
Weight:	239	219
Waist size:	42.5"	38.2"
BMI:	32.4	30
Body fat:	33.8%	27.3%
Total Pounds Removed:	20	

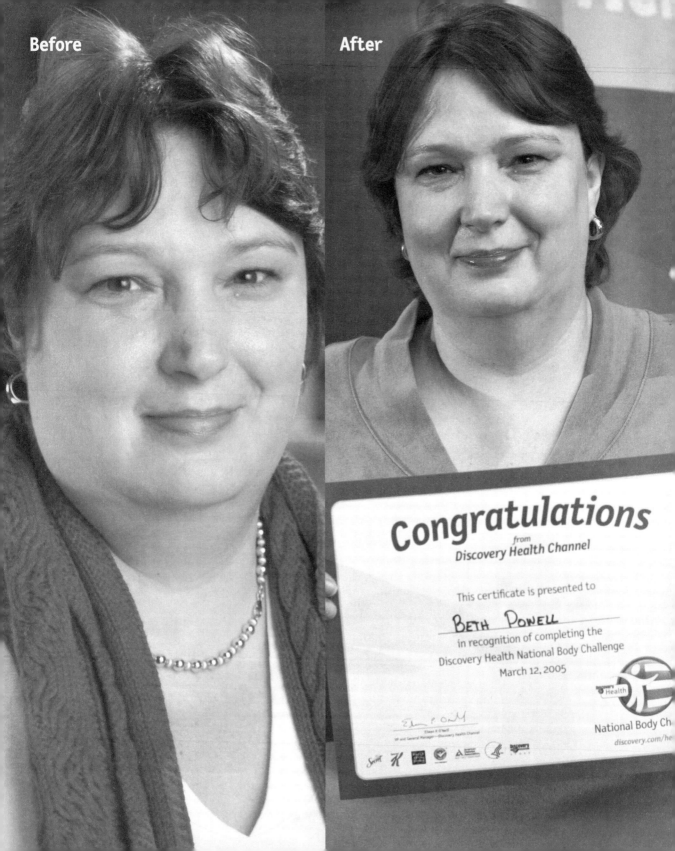

Before

After

Congratulations
from
Discovery Health Channel

This certificate is presented to

BETH POWELL

in recognition of completing the
Discovery Health National Body Challenge
March 12, 2005

Eileen K O'Neil
VP and General Manager—Discovery Health Channel

National Body Ch...

discovery.com/he...

Beth Powell
Walks *the* Talk

One winter day, Beth Powell, 45, a lobbyist for a
mental-health provider association in Washington,
D.C., went to the mall with only one goal in mind:
to buy lipstick. Instead, she stumbled upon the
Discovery Health National Body Challenge weigh-in.
Tipping the scales at 297 pounds and a survivor
of breast cancer ten years ago (with a recurrence
in 2003), Beth took the opportunity to sign up
and make some healthful changes in her life.

Beth says she wasn't a heavy kid, but admits that she tends to eat under stress. "I started gaining weight when my dad died on my birthday in 1983." When you combine the stress of her health challenges (she'd only finished a bout with chemotherapy eight months before) with a high-pressure job that has her spending a lot of time on Capitol Hill lobbying senators, as well as her age, you can see how she was a perfect candidate for the buildup of the "toxic fat" I always talk about.

All her doctors had recommended that Beth remove weight, but until the National Body Challenge, she hadn't seen any positive results. She'd tried other programs, but admits to using her calories on Fritos! It wasn't until she consulted with us that she learned about spending your calorie allotment in ways that nourish your body.

Mind

"I've had chronic insomnia for many years," says Beth. "I now sleep a lot better, and also my mood has improved." Because of her job, she's aware of all the studies about how exercise does improve moods and help combat depression, "so that's one of the things that keeps me going to the gym. I think I'm a lot more positive. I've always been outgoing—I couldn't have my job and not be—but now I feel a lot better and I have a lot more energy. It's been great for my mental attitude."

Also, her Target Motivation was to get and stay healthy in order to prevent another recurrence of breast cancer. I reminded her that obesity is a powerful risk factor for breast cancer, and every pound of excess fat she removed was saving her life. She made the connection and stuck with that focus throughout the Challenge and beyond.

Mouth

According to Beth, the hardest part of her new eating program was not having any junk carbs at night because she was used to going home and having spaghetti, or the like, for dinner. But cutting back on refined white carbs was a wise move for Beth, since recent studies have shown that they boost levels of insulin-like growth hormones linked to breast cancer. We put her on a program of 1,400 to 1,600 calories per day based upon her Resting Metabolic Rate, and she learned how to divide that up for her five meals each day: breakfast, mid-morning, lunch, mid-afternoon, and dinner. The late night, stress overeating was over.

"I've always been one to eat a lot of vegetables, so that part was fairly easy for me," she says. She also overcame her hesitancy to cook fish. "I thought I would mess it up, but I've learned how to cook it and found it's really simple and good."

Like many women, Beth didn't want to deprive herself of a little piece of chocolate every once in a while. "I bought a bag of those tiny Three Musketeers bars because they have less fat than other candy," she says. "I gave them to my neighbor and said, 'You keep them for me,' and if I go to the gym I can have one." She admits that if she had them at home, she'd eat them all. "But if I have someone who weighs 90 pounds guarding them, I'm not going to say 'give me 12.' I've got all my neighbors helping me."

Muscle

Like the other 2004 participants, Beth had to contend with blizzards during the first few weeks of the Challenge. "I'm from the South, and I really hate winter!" she says. Her solution was to utilize the resources at hand. She lives in a three-story townhouse and walked up and down the stairs to get in her cardio. She even bought some hand weights so she could do some strength training at home. "I loved the weights. I was so surprised that I did."

After the Challenge, she joined a gym close to her house and enjoys the treadmill. For inspiration, she listens to music when she works out. "It's funny," says Beth. "This shows the progression for me—the music I now listen to is so different from the music I listened to when I first started. I need more energetic music now." She rocks out to Janet Jackson on the treadmill for one and a half hours, then cycles for half an hour, and every other time does weight workouts. "It's not hard if you like it," she says.

She was also motivated by the companionship of Brian and Laura, the other participants on the Challenge. "We adored each other and still keep in touch," she says. "And I think that was key to the success of it because we were all pulling for each other."

Inspired by Beth, one of her neighbors started an exercise program, "and she'd never exercised before in her life," says Beth. "We live fairly close to each other, and she's out walking when I get home from work."

Her Proudest Achievement

Beth's proudest achievement is keeping up with her exercise. "I really didn't know that I could do it, and I never in a million years thought I would *enjoy* it," says Beth. "I'm a girly girl, and I never liked to sweat, but you know, it's not so bad!" Recently Beth attended a conference for work and went to the gym every single day while she was there. "I had to be at my conference at 7 o'clock, and I was at the gym at 5 o'clock every morning," she says. "So that's a change that will be lifelong."

Height: 5′5″		*8-Week Program*
	Before	**After**
Weight:	296.8	265.8
Waist size:	51.75″	47.3″
BMI:	49.4	42
Body fat:	53.8%	44.6%
Total Pounds Removed:		31

Her Best Tip

Be mindful. Be aware of what you put in your mouth and what it takes to burn it off. She used to eat bagels "at random," but doesn't anymore because she knows that half of one equals 30 minutes on the treadmill. Even when she chooses to have some of her old favorite, spaghetti, she's aware of portion size. Have a little, not a lot, she advises.

Her Future Plans

Beth learned healthy habits on the National Body Challenge that she plans to implement for the rest of her life. "Something has clicked," she says. She saw results from the first week of the Challenge and eventually removed 31 pounds and lowered her body fat, but knows she still has a long way to go. "I can't do it all today, and it's not going to be a straight line, but I know that I'll do it."

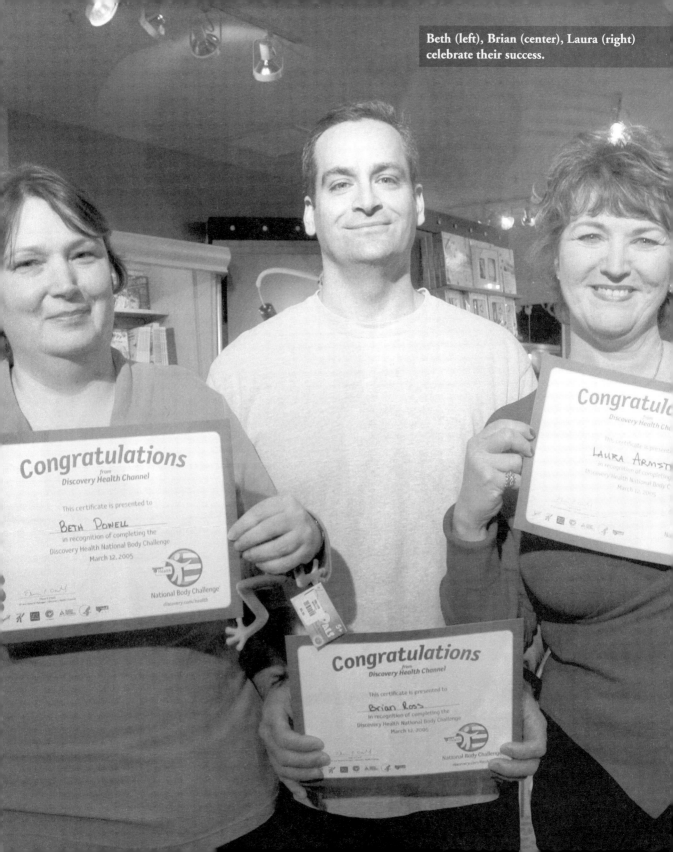
Beth (left), Brian (center), Laura (right) celebrate their success.

Before

After

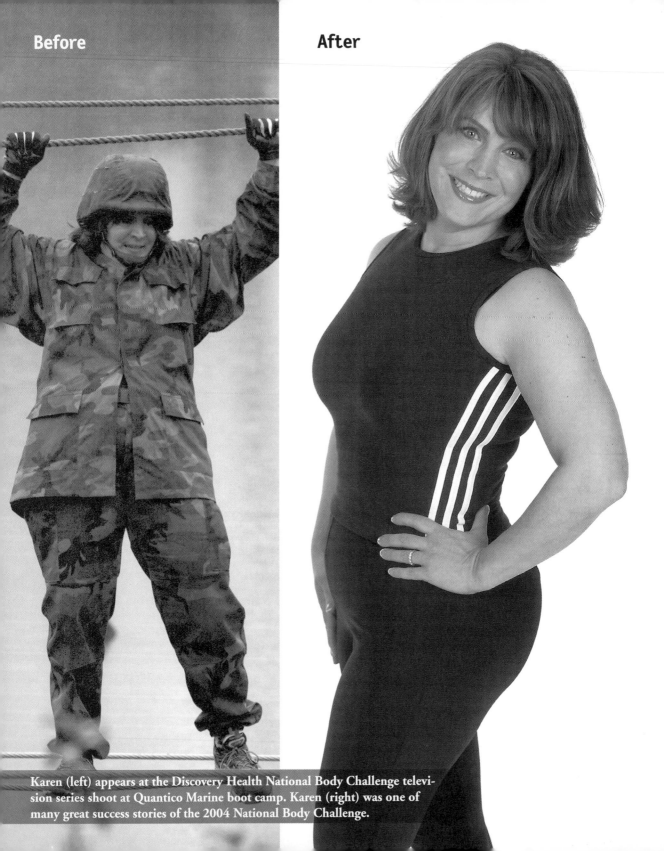

Karen (left) appears at the Discovery Health National Body Challenge television series shoot at Quantico Marine boot camp. Karen (right) was one of many great success stories of the 2004 National Body Challenge.

Karen *Staitman*
Lives *the* Sweet Life

How would you like to try removing weight while working in a cookie factory? Okay, now think about trying to remove weight while running your own cookie business *and* a candy business *and* attending trade shows full of tempting gourmet foods *and* raising three energetic kids under the age of ten. That was Karen Staitman's situation when she appeared on the 2004 season of the National Body Challenge TV series with me. Karen, 41, lives in Westlake Village, California, with her husband and three beautiful children.

At the start of the Challenge, Karen weighed in at 196 pounds and had 44 percent fat. "I was floored," she says. "I used to be a competitive figure skater, but having babies every other year and building two businesses just didn't leave much time to do anything good for me." Karen once had a slender skater's body, but after she abandoned the ice eleven years ago, she'd become, in her words, "fat and mushy." She wanted to be toned and in shape again. Now Karen was entering the peri-menopausal part of her life and knew that she needed to build back her muscle to rev her metabolism once again. She was ready for a change.

Mind

When she was carrying excess fat, Karen wore stretchy pants with stretchy waistbands all the time. "There was a period of ten years when I didn't buy clothes," she says. "My employees called me the bag lady because I wore ratty clothes with holes in them. In a sense, I was hiding. It's so much easier to wear the same clothes every day because I didn't have to think about my appearance." She would avoid going out because she had nothing to wear except outfits left over from her pregnancy.

In this respect, Karen reminds me of a woman with a similar story who, in response to my question "What size are you presently?" answered unabashedly "Elastic." When this happens, you're floating mindlessly, with no belt or waistband to keep you in tow.

Karen was also hit-and-miss about going to the beauty salon for those ten years. "When you're a busy mom, wife, and business owner, somehow you get lost in the shuffle. Couple that with being overweight and you don't want to go anywhere where the 'pretty people' are." This pattern of self- abandonment and dissociation is a familiar pattern among over-weight men and women alike.

Now consider this entry from her National Body Challenge journal: *Yesterday I did something for me—a first step—I colored my hair. Today I felt a bit like the old me: sexier, leaner, a bit blonder, and great!*

Karen's physical changes have continued to promote a new self-image. "When I'm dressed and looking good, I feel different, and then, of course, people respond to you differently," she says. Right after the Challenge when she was out shopping and wearing one of her new outfits, two girls approached her and asked if she worked in the fashion business. "I said no and asked why," Karen recounts. They told her she looked so beautiful and well put-together they were sure she did. "And that was really the nicest complement I'd ever received," she says. "I wasn't on the outside looking at something I wanted to be; I was actually being that person." She says that she also appreciates being able to go places with her children and feel good about herself.

Speaking of children, Karen is acutely aware that her Target Motivation to keep her focused on self-care is all about being there for her kids. She wants to teach them healthy habits and is creative about finding ways to get out and be active with them. In addition, she involves them in the grocery shopping decisions as well as food preparation. She's realized that her children won't be healthy unless she and her husband—who's in great shape—teach their kids by example.

Mouth

Karen's biggest challenge meant dealing with her sugar habit. "I love sugar," she says. "I'm surrounded by it every day." She'd find herself "nibbling on things—a little candy here, a cookie there." When she started to keep score, those little nibbles were adding up to over 1,000 calories a day. For the Challenge, she cut out all sugar. "I needed to start somewhere, and that was my problem—not the bread or the fat. I had withdrawals, a headache for four days straight. But after that, I was pretty good." Giving in to her cravings during the National Body Challenge would have serious consequences, so she stayed sugar-free throughout.

Now she's back eating some sugar, but she's doing it with awareness and in measured amounts. Often when she wants a little something sweet, she'll have a diet soda; other times it will be ten chocolate chips. Eating a little here and there is fine; doing it every day in large quantities is not. Fitting in her 1,400 to 1,600 calories per day was easier once she had a plan in place to have the healthy foods available throughout her busy day.

Before the National Body Challenge, Karen never ate breakfast. She was too busy to eat, and often didn't have her first meal until two in the afternoon. She was smart to start: Eating breakfast is one of the most power predictors for being successful in this lifestyle change.

Karen has also taken to heart my warning that if you fail to plan, plan to fail. "Every week I go to the market and put safe food into the rcfrigerator at work," she says. "If you go out with friends for fast food or just grab something quick, you're often not aware of what you're eating. I don't really plan my meals—I'm more of a fly-by-the-seat-of-my-pants kind of girl—but I have safe foods, so if I need anything, it's there." She keeps fruit, yogurt, and low-fat cheeses on hand.

Even during the week of last Valentine's Day, the most hectic time of her year when she works 18 to 20 hours a day, Karen did plan out meals for the whole week. In the past, she would have grabbed a cookie or a handful of candy without a second thought. But with a refrigerator full of healthy snacks and meals, "I made it through," she says.

Muscle

"The only time I ever maintained my weight was when I was skating six hours a day and running another two," says Karen. In recent years, she had become sedentary—sitting at a desk all day and crashing by 8:30.

We put her on a program of weight training three times a week and cardio for 30 minutes every day to help counter her slowing metabolism. She also mixed it up with martial arts classes, Tae Bo, and even got back on skates and loved it! "I had to learn how to skate again," she says. "I was 60 pounds heavier, so my center of gravity was off. My butt was bigger, my boobs were bigger, and nothing was quite in the same place, so I had to relearn balance."

Then, too, she met with the other competitors every few weeks to take part in Challenges and to weigh in. They climbed to the top of the Space Needle in Seattle, ran a 5K race in Houston, and competed in a triathlon in Atlanta. "It was all a lot of fun, and even though we were competing against each other, we were also cheering each other on," she says.

Karen still works out three to seven days a week. "What makes me enjoy my workouts now is music," she says. "For me it's musical theater. It just makes me go; without it I can't take one step." She really enjoys Spinning and the stair machine. "I happen to love that; it makes me sweat more than anything," She also does strength training and core work with a stability ball.

Her Proudest Achievement

Karen was recognized in the 2004 National Body Challenge for the weight she lost and her health accomplishments. She won because she had the most daunting life stresses and struggles—mother, spouse, owner of two businesses—and she managed to make a striking turnaround in her lifestyle. This wasn't a numbers game. She didn't remove the most weight—the three men all removed more. And with her 28.5 pounds of weight removal, she only squeaked by the other women by one pound. "But I was 10 years older and I had kids," she says. "I had a lot more on my plate." Karen, in fact, was a great example of meeting the challenge to become fit and healthy when you have everything coming at you.

Her Best Tip

Keep it honest. "You have to be responsible to yourself; you won't attain your goal without being honest," she says. What kept her honest was writing everything down each day. "And trust me," she says, "I'm not someone who writes down anything; I keep it all in my head. In the past that has always been my downfall." She's right, of course. You think you know what you're doing, but things happen during the day that you forget about, and they add up.

Her Future Plans

Karen says that she has small goals. "To keep exercising every day is a big thing for me to do," she says. "So my big plan is to stick to my daily plans," she says. She's going to continue eating healthfully and watching her portions. "If I get through each day, I will eventually achieve my big goal, which is to remove more weight." Karen would like to remove another 27 pounds. And while doing so, she'll continue to be the best example of healthy living to her children. After all, her most important future plan is to simply be there for them as they grow up.

Height: 5'4"		*12-Week Program*
	Before	**After**
Weight:	*196*	*167.5*
Waist size:	*38"*	*32.5"*
BMI:	*33.7*	*29*
Body fat:	*44%*	*38%*
Total Pounds Removed:	*28.5*	

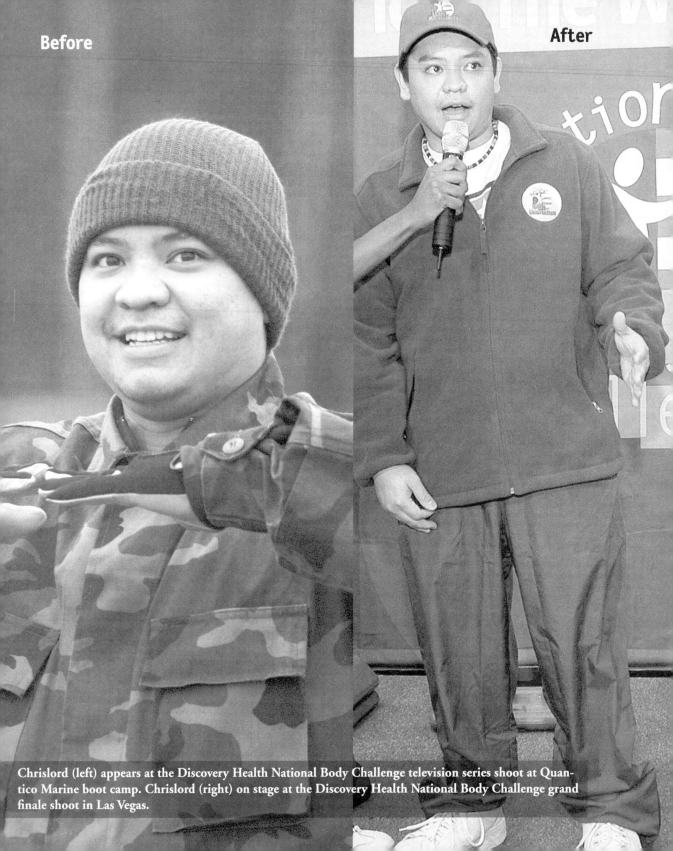

Before

After

Chrislord (left) appears at the Discovery Health National Body Challenge television series shoot at Quantico Marine boot camp. Chrislord (right) on stage at the Discovery Health National Body Challenge grand finale shoot in Las Vegas.

Chrislord Templonuevo Is Surfing *the* Wave *of* Success

When 27-year-old Chrislord Templonuevo looks back on his motivation for signing up as a participant for the 2004 National Body Challenge television series, he realizes he needed to save his own life. He lived in Houston at the time (one of the fattest cities in America), had a fairly sedentary job, and lived at home with his parents. To change his young life, he had to start with his lifestyle.

At 5'6" and weighing 202 pounds, Chrislord was a heart attack waiting to happen—and he knew it. "I want to live as long as I can and I know it's not going to happen when I'm so obese," he said at the time. So he slugged it out for 12 weeks and, 49 pounds later, he's the man he always dreamed of being, capable of doing anything he wants and feeling confident enough to push the envelope and explore the world. Explore he did! Chrislord was so energized after finishing the National National Body Challenge that three months later he packed up his bags, bid his family a fond farewell, and moved to Honolulu where he lives today. Not only has Chrislord maintained his amazing fitness achievement, but today he's out there living his dreams.

One particular passion Chrislord is living is as a hip-hop dance instructor. He also just finished his first major race, the eight-mile Great Aloha Run. His photographs, radiating health and happiness against a Hawaiian backdrop, have warmed our hearts at the Peeke Performance Center. He's literally come full circle.

Mind

For Chrislord it was all about knowing that he'd hit rock bottom. Mentally and physically, he just didn't feel like he was living life to the fullest. He couldn't keep up with guys his own age and felt socially withdrawn. He had ripe memories of kids and colleagues teasing him as he grew up. Surrounded by mental pain and disappointment, he wanted happiness and knew he'd have to fight for it.

Once he removed the 49 pounds, Chrislord kept the 2004 Discovery Health Channel National Body Challenge TV series DVD to remind him of his before picture. It didn't work for him to concentrate on his current great physical fitness. "I need constant reminders of where I will end up if I stray too far off my healthy lifestyle," he says. "I never ever want to go back there again."

Chrislord's geographic change was a necessary element to his success as well. "I couldn't stay fit in Houston," he says. "So I went from one of the fattest cities to one of the fittest when I moved to Honolulu. It's tough when you live in a city where they don't wear shirts 90 percent of the time!"

Mouth

Being part Spanish and part Filipino, Chrislord had his challenges when it came to food. After we'd measured his Resting Metabolic Rate, we determined he needed to stick to about 1,800 calories per day to achieve his goal. But he lived at home and had to struggle with late dinners as well as the typical meals prepared by his mom, which were heavy on rice and starches as well as cheeses, noodles, and beans—and large portions to boot. Also Chrislord was a sugaraholic. "Man, I could eat piles of cookies, candies, and snacks," he says. Patiently, he weaned himself off these foods and concentrated on whole foods. His family supported him all the way, and made substantial changes at home as well.

Throughout the National Body Challenge, Chrislord was amazed at how little he really understood about nutrition. "I had no idea how much I should eat. I was stunned when someone showed me a normal portion size. I'd been eating enough for a family of 12," he says.

Muscle

"The first time I had to do simple pushups and sit-ups with my National Body Challenge trainer, I couldn't believe how hard it was," says Chrislord. "That was so humbling." But he didn't feel defeated. He just kept at it consistently, blending his daily cardio activities with strength training two to three times a week. After the first few weeks, he felt good enough to start doing the one thing he loved more than anything else: hip-hop dancing. "I love it. It makes me feel alive and I also love to share that with others," he says. His 12 weeks of training paid off when, on his last show for the National Body Challenge, he danced for the camera and had all of the participants going at it with him. Chrislord had come alive!

His Proudest Achievement

For Chrislord it was achieving and then sustaining his weight removal. "It's about waking up and feeling good about myself, inside and out," he says. Good enough, that is, to share his gift for dancing with others. "There's no way I was going to be a dance instructor and not look the part. I want to inspire others and I have to do it with my own example."

His Best Tip

Never think this is over. "It's is a lifelong journey," says Chrislord. He's cautious about getting too comfortable with his new fit body, and keeps himself humbled by looking at pictures and reading recollections in his journals of what his life was once like. "Adjust your expectations from the start. You will be practicing and refining your lifestyle habits for the rest of your life. Don't even think about short term fixes. They don't exist. Get ready to work it—for you."

His Future Plans

Chrislord is young and he wants to embrace every day with the high energy and vigor of his youth. "I want to be more active in my outdoor life," he says. "I live in Hawaii and I want to try just about everything: parasailing, surfing, hiking. I can't believe I'm a runner now. I never want to lose this feeling. I'm really living my life now." Amen, Chrislord. Your energy is contagious!

Height: 5'6"		12-Week Program
	Before	After
Weight:	207	161
Waist size:	42.5"	33"
BMI:	33.3	26
Body fat:	28.7%	17%
Total Pounds Removed:	46	

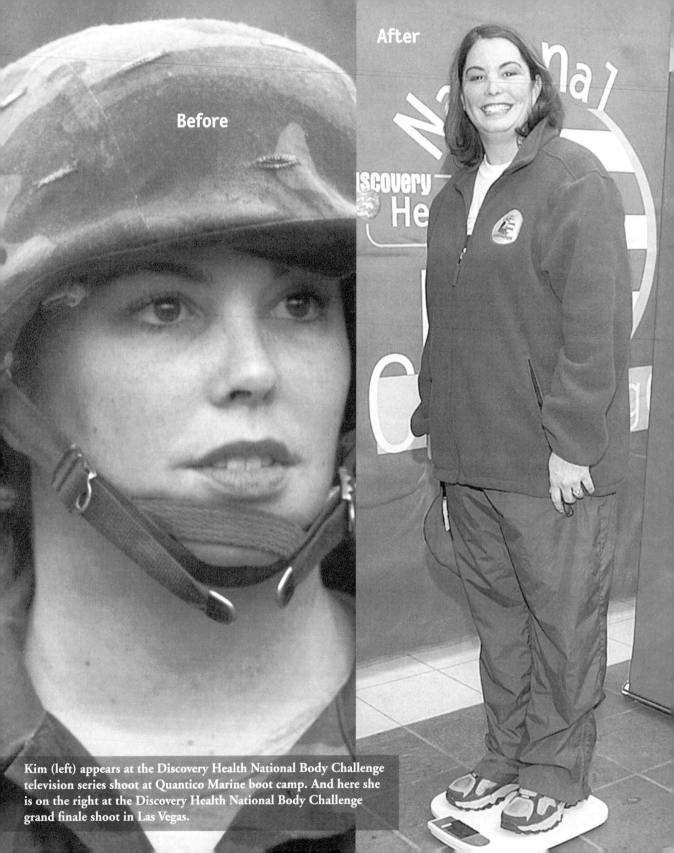

Before

After

Kim (left) appears at the Discovery Health National Body Challenge television series shoot at Quantico Marine boot camp. And here she is on the right at the Discovery Health National Body Challenge grand finale shoot in Las Vegas.

Kimberly Dontje Is
One Hot Mama

Kimberley Dontje of Atlanta was 30 and had been a flight attendant with American Airlines for ten years when she became one of our 2004 National Body Challengers. For seven of those years, she'd been flying internationally, and that lifestyle can take a toll on your health. "There were days when I would work nights and sleep through the day and then vice versa," says Kimberly. "And I'd be in cities five or six hours ahead of us and then have to come home and readjust—it was difficult."

When she was home, she says, "You couldn't get me out of the house. I was exhausted and slept ten to eleven hours daily. I'd classify myself as a couch potato." Plus, there was all that airline and airport food! It's little wonder, then, that Kimberly went from being "ridiculed for being too skinny" in college, to putting on excess weight over the years.

Mind

"It really all caught up to me when I was 28," recalls Kimberly. She and her husband wanted to have a baby. "We were successful in getting pregnant, but unfortunately I had a miscarriage. After that the pounds just came on rapidly," she says. Life became about helplessness, hopelessness, self-doubt, and punishment. "Doctors have told me that miscarriages happen all the time and there wasn't anything necessarily that I could have done to prevent it," she says. "But as a woman, that's very hard to swallow." She convinced herself that her unhealthy lifestyle was preventing her from getting pregnant. Like many stressed women, she turned to food. "I just ate and ate whatever I wanted and continued the self-destructive pattern." There were consequences: Her weight peaked at 178 pounds, and her blood pressure and cholesterol were high.

In the two years between the miscarriage and the National Body Challenge, Kimberly tried to convince herself to settle for being overweight. Nevertheless, "I would complain all the time to my friends and family, and they would encourage me, giving me suggestions of things I could do," she says. "My friends would get together and go rollerblading in the park, and I would just watch. I was embarrassed that I couldn't keep up with everyone my own age, so I chose just to sit out and make jokes about it."

The turning point came when her husband read about the National Body Challenge and tactfully approached her. "Obviously, I was very sensitive," she says. "He said, 'I love you big or small or anything in between, but I know you're not happy with yourself and this is something that maybe would really help you kick-start a new lifestyle.' So I thought, *What do I have to lose?*" She applied and was accepted. "I decided I was going to give it my everything," says Kimberly. It had taken her a while, but Kimberly was about to regroup. And her greatest Target Motivation was to be as healthy as she could for a future pregnancy and family.

Mouth

The hardest part of my Mind, Mouth, and Muscle template for Kimberly was eating less. "Right before the Challenge, my husband and I ate similar portions," she says. "The biggest challenge for me was cutting my calories and eating foods that were healthy but that would fill me up." In the beginning, it was hard to differentiate appetite and hunger and when to eat, but once she started eating appropriate portions, "my body got used to it, and that really helped." She averaged about 1,500 calories per day and found that it kept her from overeating at meals.

Kimberly says that one of the best pieces of advice her Atlanta-based trainer, Celeste, gave her was to go to bed with no food in her stomach to burn more calories throughout the night. "Not starving, obviously, but not full and having just eaten something," says Kimberly. "That seems so weird, but it worked; it truly did." Not that it was easy at first. "I was a big snacker—my husband and I would watch movies and I'd eat popcorn."

At the beginning of the National Body Challenge, they would try to eat dinner early and go for a walk. Also, "I would go to bed earlier and get up earlier, and that way I wasn't as tempted to snack," says Kimberly. She did (and still does), though, indulge as a reward for an entire week of healthy eating. "For me it's biscuits and gravy," she says. "I only allow myself to have it once a week, typically for breakfast on the weekend, 'cause I just love my biscuits! If I completely deprived myself of everything, I wouldn't sustain the program." But when she does have treats, she eats much smaller portions. She's learning the fine art of tasting!

Muscle

Kimberly freely admits that she used to hate to exercise. "I would always be out of breath, and I never continued with anything long enough to where I was reaping the benefits," she says. "I'd start doing a little bit and get the muscle soreness and then I'd give up." But the support of the National Body Challenge staff, the thought of being on television, and the help of her family and friends helped her overcome her exercise aversion. To her surprise, she loved the classes her trainer introduced her to at the gym. She also started roller skating and took swing dance lessons with her husband.

And for this woman who initially loathed exercise: "Coming in third in the 5K run on the National Body Challenge TV series was probably my proudest moment." Kimberly's goal was to be in the top three. Heck, the first and second places went to the men, as expected. So, of the women, she's the one who excelled and surprised herself with her athletic achievement. "I accomplished that, and it truly made me believe that no matter what, if I set my mind to it I could do it. And that helped me push myself even harder."

To keep herself motivated after the Challenge, Kimberly scheduled something athletic every month. "In May I did a 5K run and another in June, July was my first-ever 10K, and in August I did an all-woman triathlon," she says. After that, oh, yes … she got pregnant.

Her Proudest Achievement

Her beautiful, healthy baby girl born May 20, 2005, is Kimberly's proudest achievement. "I did everything to get in shape, and I lost another ten pounds after the National Body Challenge was over," says Kimberly. Her total was 36 pounds removed. "No matter what anybody tells me, I truly believe that getting my body ready and cleaning my system of the fat and unhealthy foods really helped me to achieve that goal."

Her Best Tip

Find your niche. "If you're somebody who doesn't like to exercise, which certainly was the case for me before the Challenge, find something that you enjoy," says Kimberly. She advises that rather than just going along with whatever your spouse or family or friends are doing, "find something just for you." She was stuck in the mind-set that the best way to remove weight was to run.

"But for me it's not," she says. "I found that I truly enjoyed kickboxing. I found one class that I absolutely loved. And there was the roller skating that I really enjoyed." Plus, she took swing-dancing lessons that included getting flung around by her husband. It's not only so much fun, but there's less to fling around of her lately!

The same advice goes for eating. The key to Kimberly's success was making the right food choices for her. Some of the foods recommended on the program didn't tickle her taste buds. "I don't like salads with oranges and apples!" she says. But she did enjoy having a whole-wheat English muffin for breakfast and likes eggs and low-fat cheese and vegetables such as peppers so she was able to find substitutions that appealed to her. "It's not going to be a lifestyle change for you if you can't find your own niche," she stresses. That's the beauty of the National Body Challenge program—you can customize and individualize the Mouth and Muscle elements to suit your unique lifestyle needs. Kimberly is living proof.

Height: 5'4½"	12-Week Program	
	Before	**After**
Weight:	178	150.5
Waist size:	39"	32"
BMI:	30.6	26
Body fat:	42%	35%
Total Pounds Removed:	27.5	

Her Future Plans

Kimberly and her husband plan to have more children and, she says, "I want to be an active family. My own family was not physically active; we'd watch TV at night. My husband and I really want to take the kids hiking and camping and bike riding and to play tennis with them—anything outdoors as a family." She is well aware of my "see one, do one, teach one" concept. "I plan to continue this healthy lifestyle; I'm not going to sit on the couch and tell my kids that you need to go out and play. I want to provide a healthy example and really show them you can eat healthily, and you can exercise, and it can be fun, not something you dread."

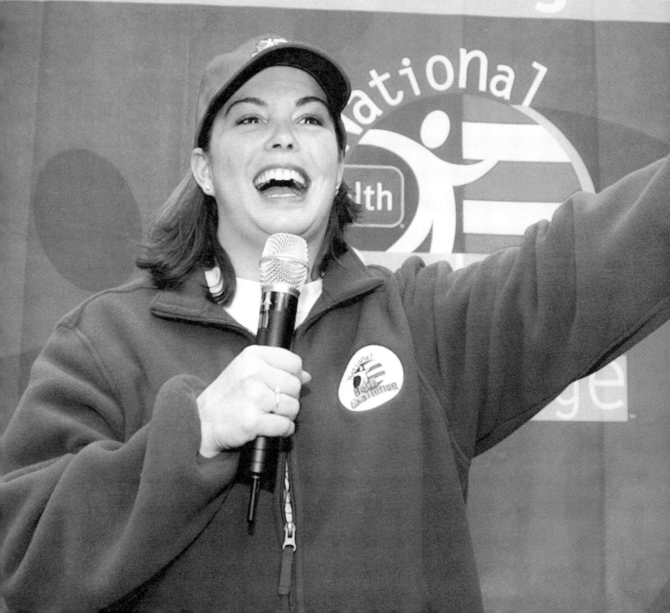

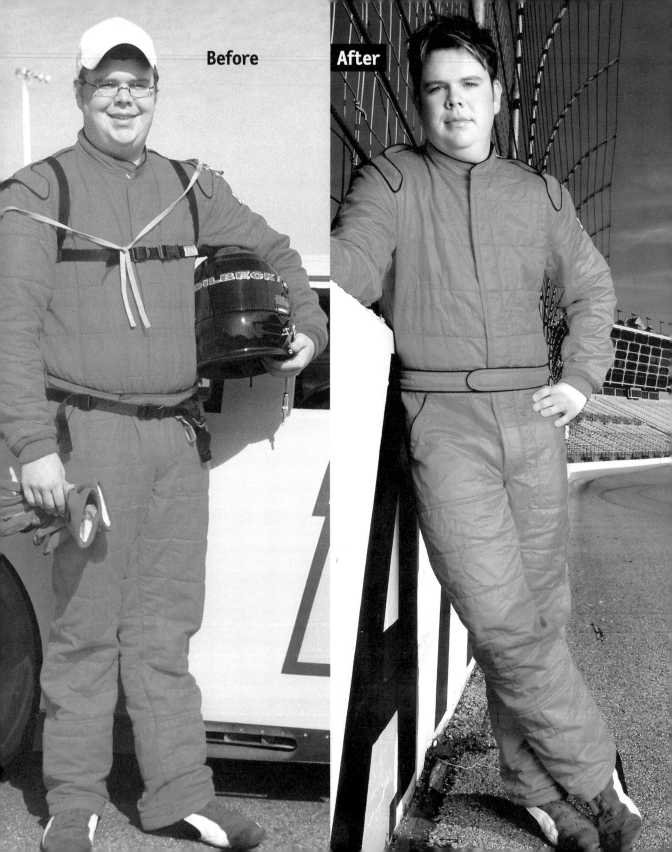

Before

After

Chris Dilbeck
Has Drive

Chris Dilbeck had a lot on his plate when he took on the National Body Challenge a year ago. He was just 18 and an entering freshman at the University of West Georgia. Additionally, he was an emerging star in the world of auto racing. "I've been racing cars since I was 12 years old, starting off with little go-carts," he says. He's now driving at one level below NASCAR and has won several state championships while placing second and third in the nation a number of times.

At the start of the Challenge, he was 220 pounds, with a goal of removing 30 pounds. "I had to work on getting in shape to make myself better in the race car," he says. The less you weigh in a race car, the faster you'll go, so in this respect, his weight was definitely holding him back. In his ambition to become a professional NASCAR driver, he's aware that being fit will not only improve his performance, but also make him more attractive to sponsors in a field where image counts. "Plus, I wanted to feel better," he says.

Mind

Chris freely admits to having had an agenda when he went on the National Body Challenge. Not only did he want to get fit, but he also wanted to take advantage of the television publicity to further his racing career. "Why not kill two birds with one stone?" he asks. "Lose weight and get some exposure for my racing. That was my thinking behind it." That's the kind of drive and motivation that makes him a winner.

"When I was younger, I played baseball," he says. "I had asthma, and the medicine they gave me had some steroids in it so it increased my appetite, and I think that's part of the reason for my being overweight. But that's no excuse. I'm sure it had an effect on my performance in sports, but I never really let it stop me."

Chris's own enthusiasm for everything he tackles is backed up by a strong support system. "All my friends that I've known since high school attend the races and hold up signs," he says. And when it came to the National Body Challenge, "my parents and my friends were behind me 100 percent," he says. "My friends would go running with me; they were just awesome—real supportive—throughout the whole thing."

Chris met his target of removing 30 pounds. "I'm just happier," he says, "and I'm proud of keeping it up."

Mouth

The Mouth part of the program was a Challenge for Chris. "It was really tough on my eating habits," he says. Those eating habits largely featured pizza! "My National Body Challenge trainer, Max, told me I was eating for four people," he says. So for him the key was to cut down on the quantity of his portions while also increasing the quality of his food. "And once I learned to do that, it wasn't that hard because I could still eat things that I wanted to." Chris and his mother had gone on various diets together, going through the classic cycle of losing ten pounds and then gaining them right back.

According to Chris, these diets failed because they were restrictive. "You would have to eat just grilled chicken, grilled chicken, grilled chicken," he says. "That would get boring to me, and that's the reason they didn't work out." Plus, he says he didn't learn anything at all about nutrition. "The National Body Challenge taught me a lot about it, and that I could have some of the foods I wanted, but just not in bulk."

He kept to 1,800 to 2,000 calories on a daily basis, spread out over four or five feedings throughout the day. He also became smarter with his snack choices and tried to make certain to eat every four hours to curb his appetite. By the end of the Challenge, he'd removed 30 pounds of excess weight and has been successful in maintaining his new weight.

Muscle

The Muscle element was more up Chris's alley. Even though he hadn't formerly worked out, he'd liked playing baseball and basketball despite not being able to always keep up with his friends. "I enjoyed the workouts because I've always done sports, and if it helps my racing, I'm all for it," he says. He had college classes in the afternoons, and then he would go to the gym to work out with his National Body Challenge trainer, Max. He discovered that "the workouts actually relaxed me." Before the Challenge, he would have trouble getting up in the morning, but then on days after he'd worked out the night before, "I could feel it in the morning. I was more energetic and ready to go." His program included lots of running and strength workouts at the gym.

After the show, Chris got even more into strength training. "And I've gained ten pounds of muscle, and dropped more fat. Everything's going well with it. I go to the gym two or three times a week, and it's just a way of life now."

He also plays football with his friends two or three afternoons a week. "I can keep up with everybody a whole lot better when it comes to running down the field," he says. "I feel that I'm more athletic, that I'm right there with them now. That's one of the main changes." He's also seen the result in his racing. "I don't get as tired during the races, and everything is just working out better."

His Proudest Achievement

Being an inspiration, Chris has heard from people all over the country. "I had an e-mail from California two days ago from someone who said they enjoyed coming to Georgia to watch me race, and they were inspired by seeing me on the TV show into losing weight as well. I've had 20 or 30 stories like that. Those people who have said I inspired them make me that much happier."

Chris did it for himself but "to know that just shedding weight and getting in shape and making it a part of your life can help other folks, too, is amazing." Oh, and by the way, inspired by Chris, his mom also removed 20 pounds. Remember, the National Body Challenge is a family affair. It's the gift that keeps on giving to everyone around you.

His Best Tip

Don't let it get you down when you first start out. "I had a really busy schedule, and that was a problem in the beginning," he says. "I was racing on Friday, Saturday, and Sunday, and then Monday through Thursday I was in class having no time for workouts, so a social life was tough." You have to make some sacrifices, he warns. "But it's going to get easier: Each time you go to the gym it gets easier; each time you go running it gets easier; each time you go to the grocery store to pick up those healthy foods it gets easier." He wants you to realize that "it's not just a little bit of change here and there; this is a full-on lifestyle change. That's the truth; that's how it is," he says emphatically.

His Future Plans

"My goals right now are to try and tone up and gain some more muscle," says Chris. He particularly wants to strengthen his lower back and neck because they're crucial during those long races. "You're sitting in a seat for a long time holding yourself up, so your lower back has to be strong." To that end, he's continuing to work with Max. He also wants to work on endurance. "I'll run for 30 or 40 minutes on the treadmill, and that helps me each and every time," he says.

Height: 5'11"		12-Week Program
	Before	**After**
Weight:	220	189
Waist size:	36"	34"
BMI:	32	26
Body fat:	32%	23%
Total Pounds Removed:	31	

Chris gets measured after
completing the Challenge.

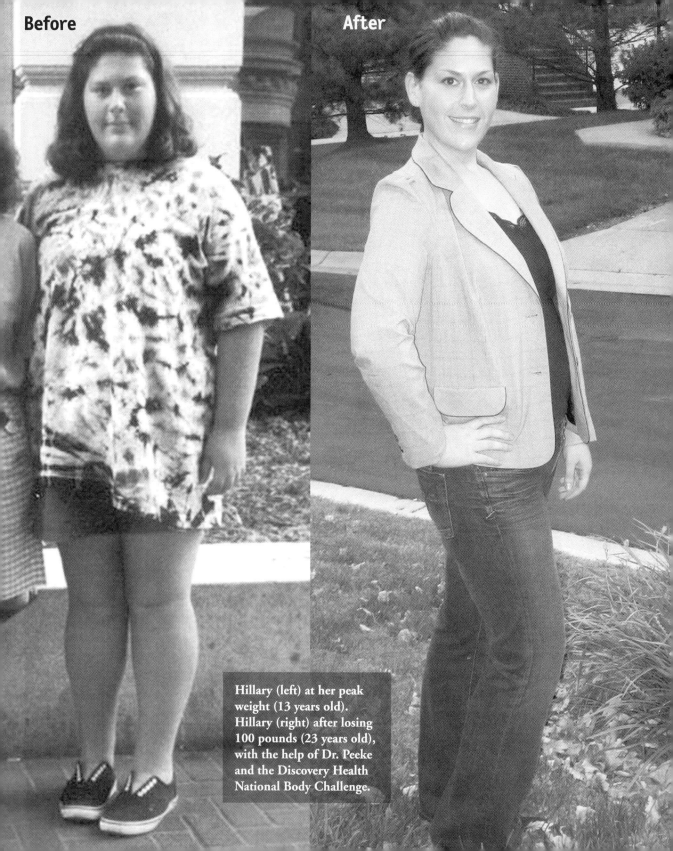

Before

After

Hillary (left) at her peak weight (13 years old). Hillary (right) after losing 100 pounds (23 years old), with the help of Dr. Peeke and the Discovery Health National Body Challenge.

Hillary Buckholtz Is a Whiz Kid

Hillary Buckholtz did the National Body Challenge to ramp up her intensity—she was actually a veteran of my Mind, Mouth, and Muscle approach. She was just 13 years old and 80 pounds overweight with high blood pressure and suffering from constant fatigue when I first met her. She had grappled with weight, food, and body-image issues pretty much for as long as she could recall.

Her mom had similarly struggled with her weight all through her own childhood, so she was familiar with getting teased, constantly dieting, and having a poor self-image. Out of compassion and love and not wanting Hillary to go through all that, she sent her daughter to various doctors, nutritionists, and therapists in an effort to address the situation. "However, being a little girl and, in retrospect I now understand not ready or prepared to fight that fight, I had a real battle," says Hillary. "And so the more focus was put on my weight and my eating, the more I'd try to take back control by going out of my way to sneak food." One of her doctors wrote in her medical file that she was a "difficult case."

This "difficult case" is now a confident 25-year-old woman who works as a fitness specialist, passionate about teaching people the benefits of healthful eating and physical activity. This once 300-pound girl is now, "normal, fit, and healthy." She also appreciates the opportunity to have an impact on others by sharing her story. "The miracles of this journey are still very present in my life," she says.

Mind

Hillary's early childhood eating problem compounded when she was ten years old. Her brother was injured in a serious car accident and had an extended stay in the hospital. "My parents were very stressed, and the family was in crisis," she says. "My memories of that period are of spending a lot of time alone, seeking comfort from the hospital vending machine." Hillary discovered that once you learn a certain survival mechanism, it becomes a dominant theme. "And so as I grew into my adolescence, I continued to go to food for comfort."

Despite this, Hillary was no wallflower. "I overcompensated by being the center of attention," she says. "I would make you laugh and entertain you before you had the opportunity to say anything negative about me. So I was popular and well liked." But that tactic no longer worked as she hit her teenage years. "I noticed that my friends were beginning to date boys and do activities that I couldn't participate in," she says. "It was becoming apparent to me that I was not one of the group, and I was starting to feel isolated."

That's when Hillary asked her mother, who was my patient, to bring her to see me. "This was the summer right before I was going to high school," she says. She was now ready and willing to make a change, not wanting to enter high school obese. "Luckily, I didn't have a lifetime's worth of failure trying to control my weight under my belt," she says. "I just did whatever the heck you told me to do and it worked at that time because I was a blank canvas."

We talked a lot about becoming resilient to stress and how to regroup and adapt to different circumstances in life. "You really talked me through a lot of those things that adolescents go through," says Hillary. "In addition to being an adolescent, I was an overweight adolescent, and then an adolescent who was losing weight. There were a number of unique challenges in all that."

Most important, Hillary came to understand that some sort of negative emotion or uncomfortable situation usually preceded her engaging in self-destructive eating behaviors. "So learning how to deal with those negative emotions and uncomfortable situations was part of the growth and journey for me," she says.

Mouth

As we worked together, Hillary learned that food is fuel. "It's a loving ritual, something that you're doing for your body, and to give yourself what you need," she says. She started to reinterpret food and understand what she needed to sustain her energy level and to power her body. It was about learning through trial and error what the right foods were for her, and what she could and could not safely eat. It was also about planning, writing down what she was eating, and being accountable for it. "And for whatever reason at the time," says Hillary, "I was willing to do that because anything was an improvement over what I'd been doing before."

Still, it was difficult when she got to high school, where a lot of bonding happens around food, especially with girls. "I had a lot of slipping and falling," she says. "I just kept getting back up, dusting myself off, and trying to practice what I learned about regrouping and taking care of myself." The same pattern continued throughout college. "I wasn't immune to the 'Freshman 15.'" She laughs. She tried to keep stress overeating under control by journaling about her emotions and developing relationships with people who she could be honest with and share. "Giving up was just not an option."

Muscle

Integrating physical activity was the other key element to Hillary's success. When she first came to see me, instead of sitting in my office we'd go for walks together. "I didn't realize at the time that you were role-modeling for me," she says. "Also, these long walks fed my spirit. Being outside, connecting with nature, and connecting with people in nature laid down positive associations with moving that are still in my head. Being in nature is a really pleasant, spiritual, loving thing I can do for myself."

Over and above that, though, at first, "I wouldn't set foot in a gym," says Hillary. "I was afraid; I was self-conscious. Figuring out the role of physical activity in my life was a slow-growth thing." She fought it, but eventually she got it. "When I moved I felt better, it was the best antidepressant." And lo and behold, she now works as a group exercise instructor. "If there's someone who's having a really hard time and they want to cancel their fitness-center membership, I tell them my story; I tell them I was 300 pounds."

Her Proudest Achievement

"I don't have one achievement that I can think of in my weight journey," says Hillary. "Every single day of my life is full of challenges, and every day that I can treat myself well, maintain a positive self-image, and respond lovingly to those challenges is an achievement."

Her Best Tip

Take it one day at a time. "For me it became overwhelming when I thought that I had to solve my weight problem (a) by myself, and (b) today," says Hillary. "And that's why I avoided it for so long even though I was in a health and social crisis." It was when she learned that it was all about what she could do *today* for herself that it became less overwhelming. One day at a time adds up.

One day at a time for Hillary has now lasted 13 years. She's had some ups and downs and expects to have more, but she knows how to regroup. And she also knows that "there's no finish line. This is a marathon journey, not a sprint."

Her Future Plans

Hillary's goal is just to be able to sustain her healthy lifestyle and to do it in a "nonfanatical, real-life way," she says. She expresses concern that many people perceive removing weight as the goal: dumping those 30 pounds is the end of the journey. "For me that was where it all began," she says. "It became about me learning how to live and how to take care of myself and how to respond to the stresses of daily life in a way that didn't involve excessive food." For her that entails prioritizing. "First things first to me means integrating some kind of physical activity into my daily life and being considerate about the kinds of food that I put into my body," she says. "It's about putting good nutrition over convenience."

Height: 5'11"   *8-Week Program*

	Before	After
Weight:	203	183
Waist size:	37"	34"
BMI:	29	25
Body fat:	34%	28%
Total Pounds Removed:	20	

RESOURCES

America on the Move
www.americaonthemove.org
1-800-807-0077

American Academy of Pediatrics
www.aap.org
1-847-434-4000

American Council on Exercise
www.acefitness.org

American Diabetes Association
www.diabetes.org
1-800-342-2383

American Heart Association
www.americanheart.org
1-800-242-8721

BAM! Body and Mind for Kids
www.bam.gov

For availability in your area,
call your local cable or satellite provider.

Discovery Health Channel
www.discoveryhealth.com

Dr. Peeke and the Peeke
Performance Center
www.drpeeke.com
301-407-0467

U.S. Department of Health
and Human Services
www.hhs.gov
1-877-696-6775

IDEA Health and Fitness Association
www.ideafit.com
1-800-999-4332 x7

Kidnetics for Kids
www.kidnetic.com

KidShape
http://www.kidshape.com
1-888-600-6444

My Food Pyramid
www.mypyramid.gov

Personal Trainers:
www.acsm.org
www.ptlocator.com
www.nsca.com/trainers/locator

ACKNOWLEDGMENTS

Three years ago, the thought leaders at Discovery Health Channel wondered what would happen if they created a national campaign to improve people's health and combat the obesity crisis. Happily, thousands of Americans answered the call and stormed the Discovery mall events, signed up online, and watched our National Body Challenge TV series with fascination. I'm honored to have been there from the beginning to develop the program and to work with such an A Team of dedicated professionals headed up by Eileen O'Neill, executive vice president and general manager of Discovery Health.

Her leadership (and love of chocolate), guided us through the long hours to complete each season. Donald Thoms, vice president of production, provided inspiration and wisdom as the program evolved. Shannon Martin, Susan Campbell, and Christine Alvarez tapped multimedia channels to get the word out to families nationwide. And my sidekick and queen of the internet, Donna Engelgau, interactive executive producer, worked with me to create a comprehensive and user-friendly Web tool program for people to use as they lived the challenge. Eternal thanks to Eric Schotz's LMNO production company and the unflappable Kathy Williamson, Ruth Rivin, and their production team. And a special thanks to Dr. Lydie Hazan for helping me with the television series. I also want to thank my fitness model Rosalind Browne for showing us such great form in the exercises.

The book was a natural next step as the challenge grew. Under the watchful eyes of Reid Tracy, president of Hay House; Angela Hynes, my witty wordsmith; and Jill Kramer, my editor and bearer of deadlines, the concept became the book. I want to thank every one of the National Body Challenge participants from its inception, including those success stories featured in the book, with special thanks to Karen Staitman and her beautiful family featured in the lively, motivating photos. And, I couldn't have done this in such short order without my fabulous Peeke Performance Center family: Vinita Stone, Torne Jacobson, Rachel Hejnal, Eva Rand, Eric Eckenrode, and Shari Frishett.

Of course, none of this is possible without Amanda Urban, my fearless agent, and James Gregorio, who labored tirelessly over all things legal. Fervent thanks to my good friend and colleague Jim Hill, Ph.D., who continues to teach me what a "successful loser" is all about. My deepest appreciation to Governor Michael Huckabee and his wonderful wife, Janet, who have joined us in this national campaign as our spokespersons for all American families seeking health and wellness.

And, of course, my family, Art and Sheila Walsh, and Eliot Pearl and Aunt Eva for their ongoing love and inspiration. Finally, eternal thanks to Mark, my soul mate, for enduring the weeks of writing and filming, patiently awaiting the final "it's a wrap."

About the Author

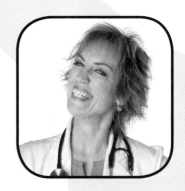

Pamela Peeke, M.D., M.P.H., F.A.C.P., is a clinical assistant professor of medicine at the University of Maryland School of Medicine, a Pew Foundation scholar in nutrition and metabolism, and an adjunct senior research fellow at the National Institutes of Health. A regular contributor to *Good Housekeeping*, Dr. Peeke is frequently quoted in *O* magazine, *Shape*, *Vogue*, *Fitness*, *More*, *Glamour*, and *Redbook*. Dr. Peeke is a member of Oprah's O Team of medical experts. She's the author of the *New York Times* bestseller *Body for Life for Women*, and the national bestseller *Fight Fat After Forty*. As chief medical correspondent for nutrition and fitness for Discovery Health Channel, she is the featured expert for the National Body Challenge Event, for which she's a national spokesperson.

We hope you enjoyed this Hay House book.
If you'd like to receive a free catalog featuring additional
Hay House books and products, or if you'd like information
about the Hay Foundation, please contact:

Hay House, Inc.
P.O. Box 5100
Carlsbad, CA 92018-5100

(760) 431-7695 or (800) 654-5126
(760) 431-6948 (fax) or (800) 650-5115 (fax)
www.hayhouse.com • www.hayfoundation.org

✦

Published and distributed in Australia by:
Hay House Australia Pty. Ltd. • 18/36 Ralph St. • Alexandria NSW 2015
Phone: 612-9669-4299 • *Fax:* 612-9669-4144 • www.hayhouse.com.au

Published and distributed in the United Kingdom by:
Hay House UK, Ltd. • Unit 62, Canalot Studios
222 Kensal Rd., London W10 5BN • *Phone:* 44-20-8962-1230
Fax: 44-20-8962-1239 • www.hayhouse.co.uk

Published and distributed in the Republic of South Africa by:
Hay House SA (Pty), Ltd., P.O. Box 990, Witkoppen 2068
Phone/Fax: 27-11-706-6612 • orders@psdprom.co.za

Distributed in Canada by:
Raincoast • 9050 Shaughnessy St., Vancouver, B.C. V6P 6E5
Phone: (604) 323-7100 • *Fax:* (604) 323-2600

✦

Tune in to **www.hayhouseradio.com**™ for the best in inspirational talk radio featuring top Hay House authors! And, sign up via the Hay House USA Website to receive the Hay House online newsletter and stay informed about what's going on with your favorite authors. You'll receive bimonthly announcements about: Discounts and Offers, Special Events, Product Highlights, Free Excerpts, Giveaways, and more!
www.hayhouse.com